JN301067

絶望のなかのほほえみ

Smile in Despair
Stories from a Cambodian AIDS ward
Goto Masaru

カンボジアのエイズ病棟から　　　後藤勝

めこん

まえがき

　初めてティーと出会ったのは2001年3月だった。

　バッタンバン州リファラル病院は市内の川沿いにある。フランス植民地時代に建てられた病院の天井はやけに高く、古くて巨大な扇風機が、頭上でゆっくりと回っていた。時折激しいスコールが降り、病室の床は雨漏りのため、いつも水浸しになっていた。

　感染病棟には無造作にベッドが置かれ、その他の設備は何もなかった。15人ほどの患者たちがいたが、動くことのできる者は中庭に出ているので、病棟内は怖いほど静まり返っていた。時折赤ん坊の泣き声が聞こえた。体が弱って動けない寝たきりの人々が、痛みを我慢しながら、じっと窓の外の景色を眺めていた。

　一番隅のベッドに、女性がひとりいて、干し終わった洗濯物を1枚ずつ丁寧にたたんでいた。ほほえみながら「私はティーよ」と言った。まるで枯れ木のように痩せ細った彼女は、とても29歳に見えない。ほとんどの患者がそうであるように、ティーもたった1人でエイズと闘っていた。

　夫は昨年エイズで亡くなったという。幼い子供が1人いて、今は祖父に預けているとも言った。

　ティーは話をしながら、時々苦しそうに咳き込んだ。エイズは免疫機能を低下させる。感染病棟にいるエイズ患者の8割が結核を患っていて、症状悪化を急速に進めて命を落とす場合が最も多かった。

　以来僕は、感染病棟を訪れるたびにティーを訪ねた。果物を食べながら語り合い、時には大部屋の角にハンモックを吊って一夜を明かしながら、僕は彼女にカメラを向けた。エイズが体を蝕み、ひどい痛みを伴う時でも、ティーは笑顔を絶やさなかった。そして日に日に、彼女の姿は変わっていった。少しずつ髪が抜け落ち、全身の皮膚が爛れはじめた頃、彼女はカンボジア人女性にとって命の次に大切な黒髪をばっさりと切った。「体力の限界がきたの。髪を洗う力もなくなったわ」

　2005年5月のよく晴れた日、ティーから、病院の中庭で写真を撮ってと頼まれた。同じ病魔と闘っている友人のテットという女性を誘い、彼女は中庭に出た。

　「昨日は隣で寝ていた女性が死んだわ。いつ死ぬかもしれないから、その前に写真を撮っておくの」ティーはか細い声で言った。彼女はきれいに化粧をして、一番のお気に入りの洋服を着ていた。

　2人並んで数枚撮影したあと、彼女はつぶやいた。

　「以前のような元気な体に戻れたら、どんなに素晴らしいでしょうね」

　ティーは「ありがとう」と言い、嬉しそうに笑うと、杖をついてゆっくりと病棟に向かって歩いていった。

　それから2ヵ月後、僕はまたリファラル病院にやってきた。

大部屋の一番隅にあったティーのベッドを見た。そこには誰もいなかった。いつも使っていたシーツもなく、ただ汚れたマットが置いてあった。友人のテットがいた。
「ティーはね、このまえ死んじゃったよ」
遺体を数日間保管して、家族が引き取りに来るのを待ったけど、結局誰も来なかったという。テットは言った。
「ティーは死ぬ前日まで、あなたのことを待っていたよ」
何も言えなかった。自然に体の力が抜けていった。「写真を撮ることの最終的な目的はあなたたちを助けること」と言った僕の言葉を、ティーは最後まで信じていた。くやしかった。何をしているのかと自身を責めた。自分を信じてくれた彼女に対して、僕はこれまでにない罪悪感を覚えた。
ティーを茶毘に付した寺院は近くにあると聞き、僕はそこに向かった。寺院の火葬場には大きなドラム缶があり、中に遺灰と共に遺骨が山積みになっていた。
「引き取り手のいない遺骨が多いのです。みな家族に見捨てられた者たちです」若い僧侶が言う。遺骨のほんの一部だけが無縁仏を供養する本堂に納められ、その他の遺灰は裏庭に捨てられている。見ると、放牧された牛が、捨てられた遺灰を食べている。
僧侶に事情を話すとドラム缶の前で線香を焚いてくれた。煙に包まれながら僕はその前で手を合わせた。他に何ができただろう。

カンボジアには今でも、ティーのような境遇の女性が多くいる。生きる希望を持ち、エイズと闘う意志があるが、みな最後には力尽きて、ひとりで死を迎えている。

病魔と闘いながら、必死で生きていたティー。絶望の時にほほえむことができる人こそ本当に優しい人なのだと、僕はティーから学んだ。懸命に生きた彼女の姿はいつまでも僕の脳裏に残る。エイズと闘い続けたティーにこの本を捧げる。

Prologue

I first met Tee in March 2001.

Battambang Referral hospital is located along the river in the center of this city in western Cambodia. The hospital, with high ceilings and huge old fans turning slowly, was built during French colonial times. Severe squalls sometimes fell, and water from numerous leaks would soak the floor in the epidemic ward.

Beds were placed simply in the epidemic ward, and there was no other equipment. There were about 15 patients, but it was very quiet, because patients who could move themselves went outside to the courtyard. I heard a baby's cry sometimes. Some patients whose bodies grew too weak would lie on their beds and stare at the scene outside the window.

I saw one woman in a bed in the corner, and she was folding her clothes beautifully.

She smiled and said to me, "I am Tee". She was as thin as a dead tree and didn't seem 29 years old. Most of the patients in the ward were fighting AIDS alone, and Tee was among them.

"My husband died from AIDS last year," she said. She also said that she had sent her little child to take care of her grandfather.

Tee coughed a lot when she talked. AIDS weakens the immune system. Eighty percent of the AIDS patients in the epidemic ward suffered from tuberculosis. Their symptoms often advanced rapidly, and that caused most patients' deaths.

Whenever I visited the epidemic ward, I went to see Tee. We sometimes ate fruit together and we talked about our lives. I sometimes slept in a hammock by her bed. Eventually, I turned my camera to her. Tee always smiled, even though AIDS spoiled her body and left her in cruel pain. Her figure changed day by day. She started to lose her hair. And when her skin became covered in sores, she cut her beautiful long black hair by herself. Long, black hair is the most important thing for Cambodian women.

I asked her why she did that and she answered, "The limit of my physical strength came. I don't even have the energy to shampoo my hair now."

One day Tee asked me to take a picture of her in the courtyard. It was a sunny day. She invited one of her friends, Tet, who was fighting the same disease, and we left for the courtyard.

"The woman sleeping in the neighboring bed died yesterday. I want to take a picture of myself because I don't know when it will happen to me," Tee said in a feeble voice.

For that photo, she wore her favorite clothes and she put on beautiful makeup. Tee muttered after I took several pictures of her,

"How wonderful if we can be returned to cheerful bodies like before."

Then, Tee smiled and said, "Thank you." She seemed to be happy. After that she walked slowly toward the ward, leaning on a stick.

Two months later, I returned to the Referral hospital. I visited the epidemic ward and saw Tee's bed in the corner. But no one was there. There was only a dirty mat and no cover sheet.

I saw Tet and she said, "Do you know? Tee, she just died recently."

After Tee died, the body was kept for several days so her family could pray over her, but no one came. Then Tet told me, "Tee waited for you. She waited for you until the day before dying."

I could not find any words. The power in my body was lost. Tee believed my words, "The purpose of taking pictures is to help you." I was filled with sadness and I asked myself, "What have I done?" I blamed myself.

I felt guilty because Tee had trusted me.

I heard that the temple where Tee's body was cremated was near the hospital. I went there. And there was a big steel drum in the crematorium, and I saw a lot of ashes piled inside. "They are the ashes which are not taken by families. They are the people deserted by their families," a young priest told me.

After a cremation, only a few ashes are delivered to the inner temple for a memorial service. The rest are kept in the steel drum before they are thrown away in the backyard. I saw a cow grazing and eating ashes that had been thrown away earlier.

I told my story of Tee to a priest, and he lit an incense stick in front of the steel drum. I put my hands together in front of the ashes, covered with the incense smoke. I only could put my hands together. And I only could do penance in front of ashes; there was nothing else I could do.

Even now, in Cambodia there are many women who endure the same circumstances as Tee. They hope to live and are willing to fight AIDS, but they exhaust their strength and they die alone.

Tee, though quiet, fought very hard against the disease. She taught me that human beings who are able to smile no matter how desperate their situation, are people with true hearts. She was eager to live, and her figure will be in my mind forever.

I dedicate this book to my friend Tee, who kept the fight against AIDS.

目次

まえがき ……………………………………………………… 01
エイズ「後天性免疫不全症候群」 ……………………… 07

1　バッタンバン州リファラル病院 ……………………… 09
2　モム ……………………………………………………… 13
3　ソフィア ………………………………………………… 18
4　リム ……………………………………………………… 22
5　イン ……………………………………………………… 25
6　ラッタナー ……………………………………………… 28
7　サオ ……………………………………………………… 31
8　サビンとリン …………………………………………… 34
9　変わりゆく首都 ………………………………………… 37
10　売られる子供たち ……………………………………… 42
11　リナ ……………………………………………………… 46
12　ミセス・コンドーム …………………………………… 51
13　カンハ …………………………………………………… 55
14　チップ …………………………………………………… 58
15　ヒム ……………………………………………………… 63
16　スセップ ………………………………………………… 71
17　セリ ……………………………………………………… 75
18　ホーン …………………………………………………… 80
19　キーロック ……………………………………………… 84
20　ティー …………………………………………………… 88

あとがき …………………………………………………… 93

Contents

Prologue ……………………………………………………… 03
AIDS "Acquired Immunodeficiency Syndrome" ………… 08

1　Battambang Referral Hospital ………………………… 09
2　Moum ……………………………………………………… 13
3　Sophea …………………………………………………… 18
4　Lim ………………………………………………………… 22
5　Ing ………………………………………………………… 25
6　Rattana …………………………………………………… 28
7　Sao ………………………………………………………… 31
8　Savin and Lin …………………………………………… 34
9　Phnom Penh Changes …………………………………… 37
10　Trafficked Children …………………………………… 42
11　Lina ……………………………………………………… 46
12　Mrs. Condom …………………………………………… 51
13　Kanha …………………………………………………… 55
14　Tip ……………………………………………………… 58
15　Hym ……………………………………………………… 63
16　Sutthep ………………………………………………… 71
17　Seri ……………………………………………………… 75
18　Horn ……………………………………………………… 80
19　Ky Lok …………………………………………………… 84
20　Tee ……………………………………………………… 88

Epilogue …………………………………………………… 94

カンボジア

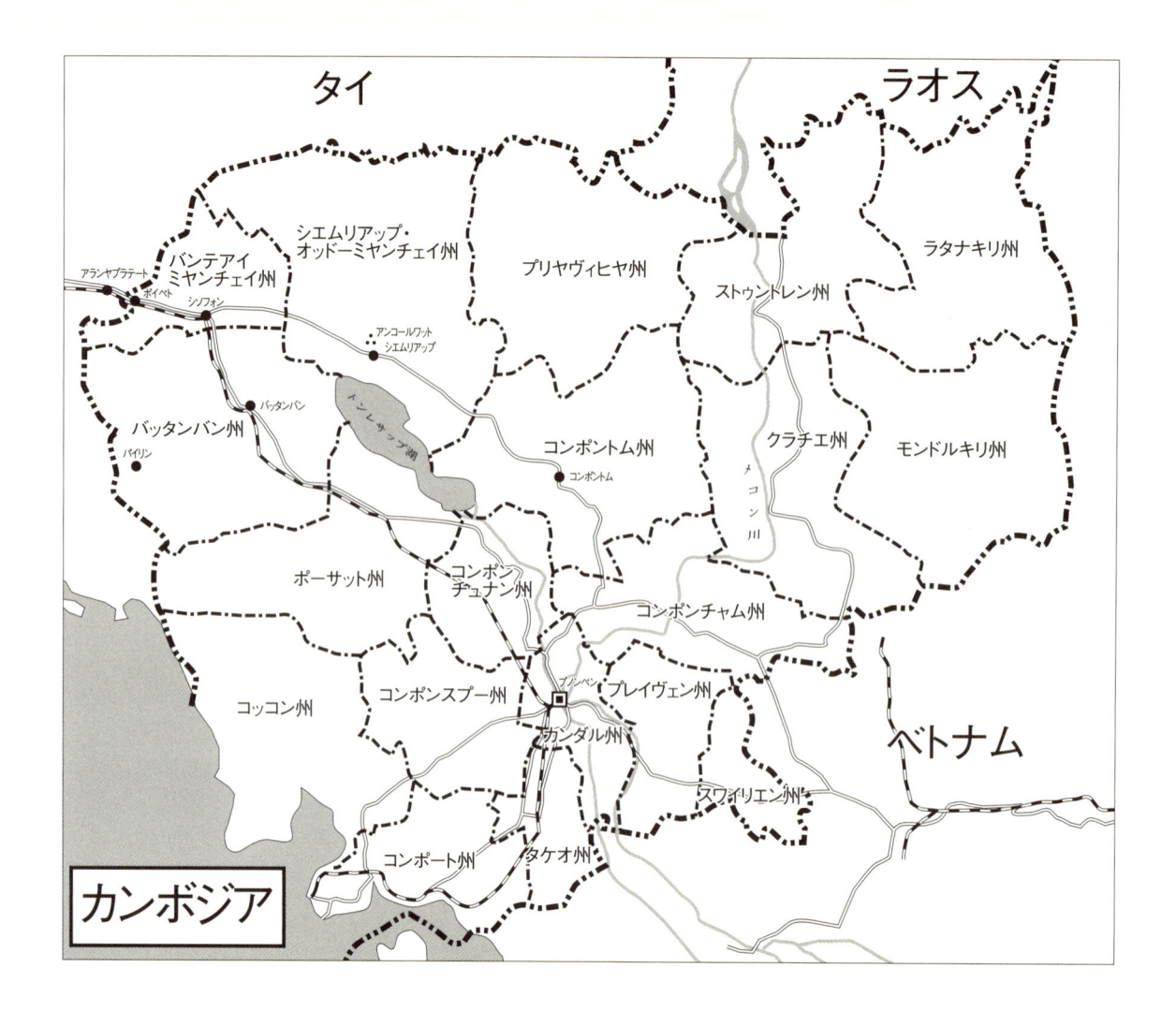

- タイ
- ラオス
- ベトナム

州

- バンテアイミヤンチェイ州
- シエムリアップ・オッドーミヤンチェイ州
- プリヤヴィヒヤ州
- ストゥントレン州
- ラタナキリ州
- バッタンバン州
- コンポントム州
- クラチエ州
- モンドルキリ州
- ポーサット州
- コンポンチュナン州
- コンポンチャム州
- コッコン州
- コンポンスプー州
- プレイヴェン州
- カンダル州
- コンポート州
- タケオ州
- スワイリエン州

都市・地名

- アランヤプラテート
- ポイペト
- シソフォン
- アンコールワット
- シエムリアップ
- バッタンバン
- パイリン
- コンポントム
- トンレサップ湖
- メコン川
- プノンペン

エイズ「後天性免疫不全症候群」

エイズは正式には AIDS「後天性免疫不全症候群」と呼ばれ、HIV（ヒト免疫不全ウィルス＝通称 HIV ウィルス）の感染によって引き起こされる病気だ。HIV に感染すると、HIV ウィルスは人間の免疫機能の中心的な役割をしているリンパ球（白血球の１種）そのものを破壊する。そして結核や肝炎などの病気に HIV 保持者が感染すると、もはや HIV に侵された免疫システムは闘うことはできない。さまざまな感染症や悪性腫瘍などを引き起こし、命を落とす確立が非常に高くなる。

1990年代後半から HIV の増殖を抑える薬剤として、タンパク質分解酵素阻害剤（PIs）やアジドチミジン（AZT）、ラミブジン（3TC）など十数種類の薬が開発されている。しかし、これらを組み合わせて服用する多剤併用（カクテル）療法は、年間１万5000ドル以上の費用がかかり、とても発展途上国の人々には手が届かない。「AIDSVAX」と呼ばれる HIV 感染予防ワクチンの開発も期待されているが、まだ臨床試験段階だ。世界中の研究者たちが今もエイズ撲滅のために研究を続けている。しかし、HIV がエイズを引き起こす正確な仕組みなどはいまだに解明されていない。

2004年、国連エイズ合同計画（UNAIDS）は25年前には未知の病だったエイズによる死者が累計で2000万人を超えたと報告した。報告書によると、2004年だけで約310万人が死亡、新たに約490万人がエイズに感染し、世界の感染者は過去最高の約3940万人と言われる。そして途上国には治療を受けなければ近い将来死亡する感染者が600万人いるが、2003年末までに治療を受けられたのは40万人にすぎなかった。

カンボジアで初めて HIV ウィルスが発見されたのは1991年である。その後国内でエイズが爆発的に広まり、94年には１日に110人が HIV に感染し、翌年には国民の70人に１人が感染者となった（国立エイズ局）。すでに2003年までの12年間で、９万4000人がエイズで死亡、このままだと2010年までに23万人の国民がエイズで死亡すると言われている（UNAIDS）。

国立エイズ局の推計では、2005年１月現在、国内の15歳から49歳までの HIV 感染者は約15万7500人。地道なエイズ教育の成果があって、HIV 感染者の数は１日20人と減少した。しかし人口1300万人のカンボジアで、現在約2.6％が HIV 感染者またはエイズ患者である（UNAIDS）。感染率はアジア・太平洋地域で最も高い。

エイズ孤児たちの問題も深刻になっている。ユニセフ（国連児童基金）によると、カンボジアで両親をエイズで失う子供たちの数は、2005年までに15万人に達すると予測されている。６万人の子供たちが現在 HIV に感染しているが、生き延びるために必要な延命薬を受けている子供たちは、たったの250人だけだ（国立エイズ局）。これまでに HIV に感染してエイズを発病した子供たちは７～８万人。しかし現在でも、実態調査が充実しておらず、明確な数字はわかっていない。

AIDS "Acquired Immunodeficiency Syndrome"

AIDS, acquired immunodeficiency syndrome, is caused by HIV, the human immunodeficiency virus.

When infected with HIV, the central role of the immune system is destroyed. A healthy immune system can restrain the HIV virus. But when HIV patients catch diseases such as tuberculosis or hepatitis, the immune system will break down and be unable to fight HIV. After that, AIDS patients are susceptible to various infectious diseases or malignant tumors, and the chances of death escalate.

Since 1990, about 10 types of medicines for restraining the multiplication of HIV have been developed. These include PIs (protease inhibitors), AZT (azithromycin) and 3TC (lamivudine). Combining these medicines, a treatment called the multiple combination or drug cocktail, costs more than 15,000 US dollars a year. Many people in developing countries are not receiving these medicines because they are so expensive.

The development of an AIDS vaccine, called "AIDSVAX," is still in the experimental stages. Researchers worldwide continue to search for ways to eradicate AIDS.

In 2004, the Joint United Nations Programme on HIV/AIDS (UNAIDS) reported that the AIDS death toll had exceeded 20 million – this, from a sickness that was virtually unknown a quarter century ago. According to the UNAIDS report, 3.1 million people died of AIDS in 2004, and 4.9 million people were newly infected with HIV. Worldwide, in 2004, 39.4 million people were infected with HIV, more than ever before.

In developing countries, 6 million AIDS patients will die in the near future if medical treatment is not given. By the end of 2003, only 400,000 AIDS patients in the developing world were receiving treatments.

The HIV virus first surfaced in Cambodia in 1991. After that, AIDS spread quickly across the country. On average, 110 Cambodians were infected with HIV each day in 1994, and by the following year, one of every 70 Cambodians was an HIV carrier (National Aids Authority).

In the 12 years since, 94,000 Cambodians have died of AIDS. If these numbers continue, 230,000 people will die of AIDS by year 2010 (UNAIDS).

According to the National Aids Authority, about 160,000 people between the ages of 15 and 49 are currently infected with HIV in this country. The number of HIV infections has decreased as a result of steady AIDS education, but still, about 20 people are infected each day. About 2.6 percent of the Cambodian population, which totals 13 million, is infected with HIV or AIDS (UNAIDS). Cambodia still has the highest infection rate in the Asia-Pacific region.

As a consequence, the problem of AIDS orphans is growing. According to UNICEF, 150,000 children are expected to lose parents to AIDS by 2005. About 60,000 children are infected with HIV, but only 250 children receive necessary life-sustaining medicine (National Aids Authority). Up until now, numbers show that 70,000-80,000 children have been infected with HIV. But research is incomplete and no one knows the exact number of victims.

1　バッタンバン州リファラル病院

　2001年3月。内戦後のカンボジアを取材するために、バッタンバン州リファラル病院を訪ねた。病院の建物は年々老朽化し、塀が所々崩れ落ちている。中庭の広場では、木陰のベンチに座った患者たちが、思い思いに時間をつぶし、広場では子供たちが無邪気に遊んでいた。

　しばらくして雨雲が見え、滝のようなスコールが降り始めた。感染病棟は雨漏りがひどく、床は水浸しになっている。錆びたベッドが20ほど置いてあり、この日患者は16人いた。白衣を着た看護師が1人いて、忙しそうに動き回っている。

　「今エイズ末期患者が6人います。既に免疫力が極度に落ち、このままだと、みな数ヵ月以内に死んでしまいます」

　どこからか低いうめき声が聞こえた。病室の一番角のベッドに、全身を蚊帳で包んだ1人の男性が座っていた。壁を見つめながら、独り言を言い、時折大きな声で唸る。エイズが原因で、脳に障害ができたという。付き添いの家族はおらず、その横には痩せた女性が静かに横たわっていて、天井をじっと眺めていた。

1 Battambang Referral Hospital

In March 2001, I visited Battambang Referral hospital while covering the story of Cambodia after its civil war. The building was already so old that some of its walls had collapsed. Outside, patients sat on a bench in the shade of a tree, killing time, while in the courtyard children played innocently.

　I saw a rain cloud build over a short time. Soon, a squall began to drop like a waterfall. In the epidemic ward, the roof leaked severely, and water soaked the floor. There were about 20 rusty beds and 16 patients on this day. One nurse in a white coat was moving around, and seemed to be busy. "Now six terminal AIDS patients are in the ward. Their immune systems have already fallen excessively; if conditions continue the same, they will die within a few months."

　I heard a low groan from somewhere. One man had wrapped his whole body in a mosquito net, and he was sitting on a bed in the corner of the epidemic ward. He muttered and chanted; sometimes he groaned loudly while facing the wall. A nurse said that his brain was damaged by AIDS. Next to him, a thin woman lay quietly on her side, looking at the ceiling. There was no family to take care of either of them.

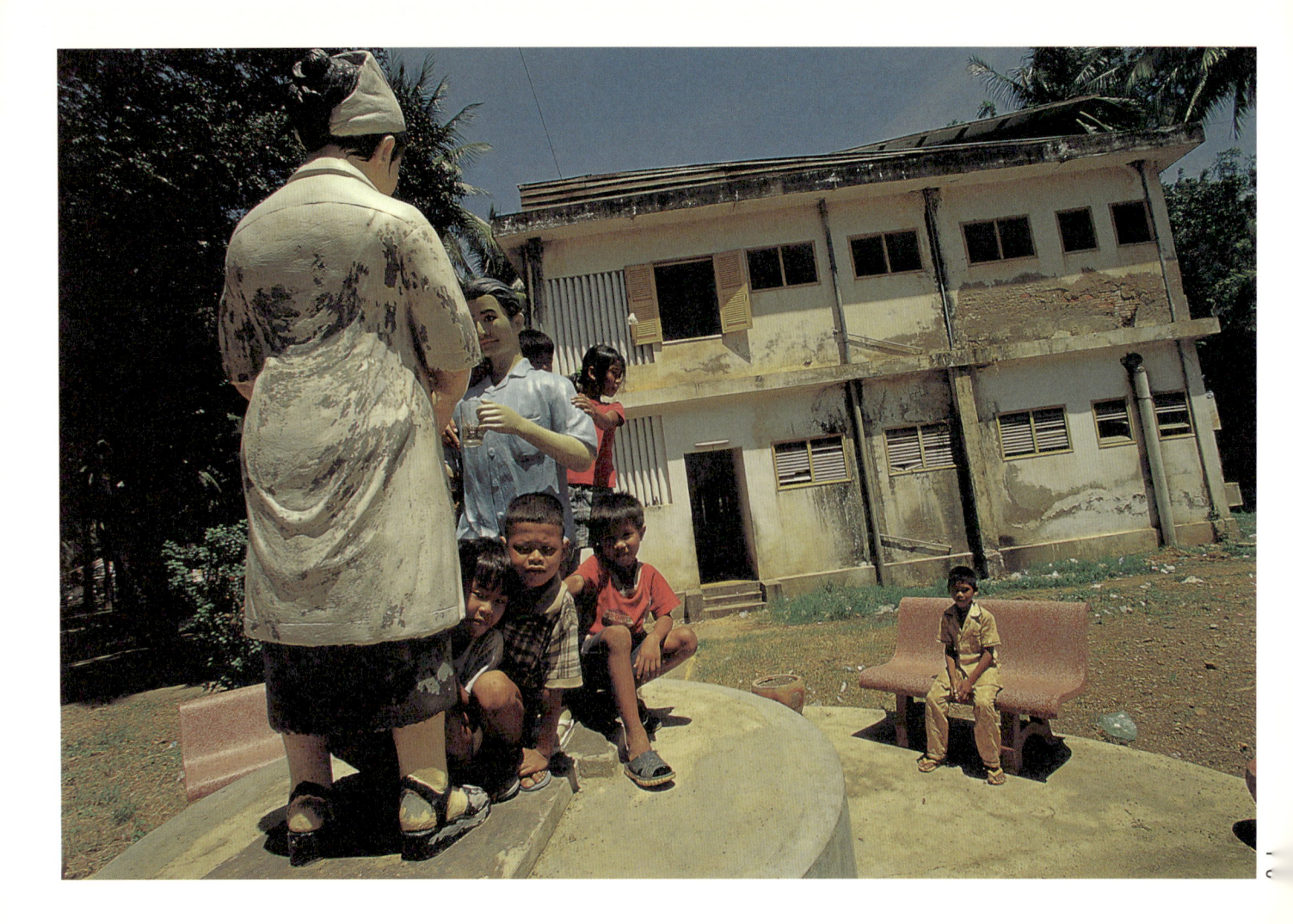

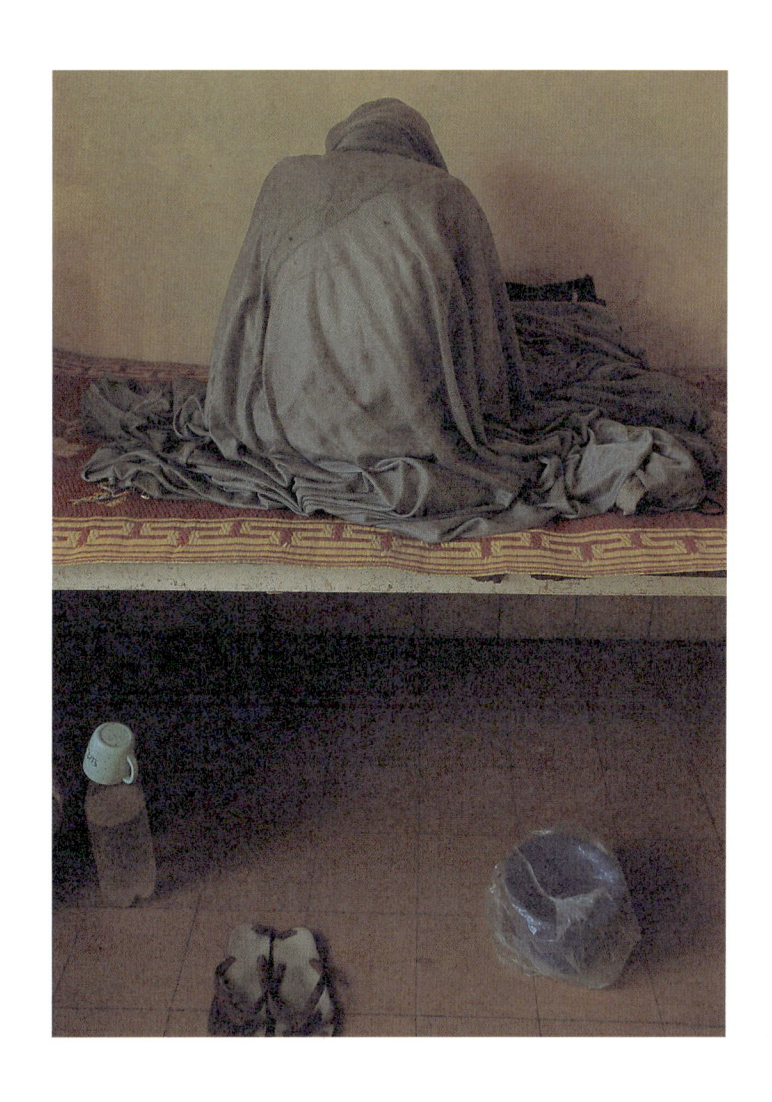

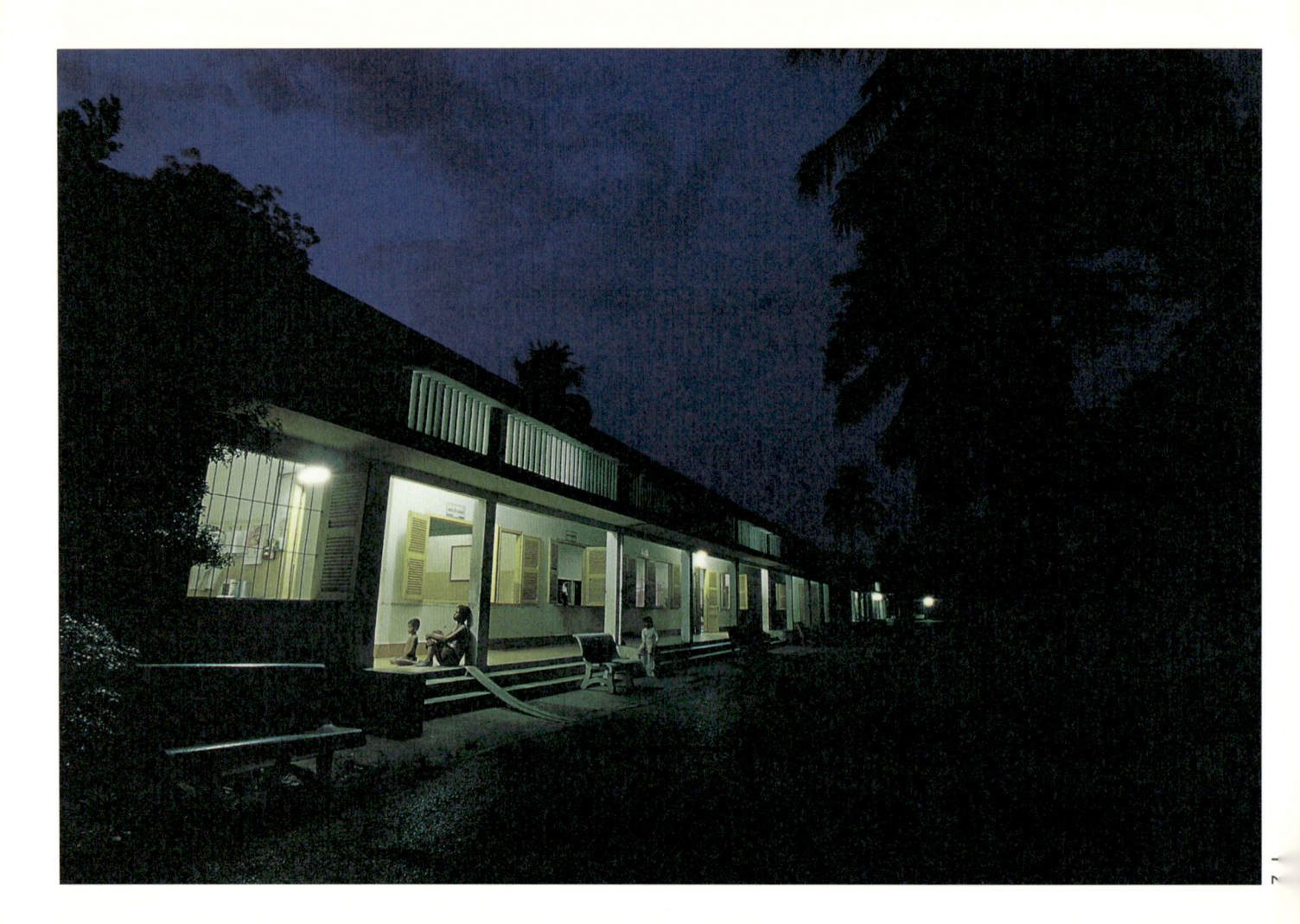

2 モム

　2002年8月。薄暗い病室で1人の女性が娘にお粥を食べさせていた。28歳になるモム。まるで老婆のように痩せ衰えている。

　彼女は汗を吸って汚れたシャツをまくり上げた。あばら骨が浮き出て、骨と皮だけになった彼女の体を見て、僕は言葉をなくした。

　「体がこんなに痩せてしまった。体に火がついたように、ずっと火照っている。このまま私は灰のように枯れてしまうのかしら」

　写真を撮るべきかどうか、迷った。カメラバッグを肩から下ろし、窓の外の景色に目を向けた僕に彼女は言う。

　「ほら、私の写真を撮りなさい」

　僕はカメラを持ち、ファインダーを覗いた。そこには痩せて生気を失った女性の姿があった。彼女はため息をつき、小さく声を上げた。

　「早くこの苦しみから逃れたい」

　モムに死が訪れたのは、それから1ヵ月後だった。死の数日前、彼女は自ら娘を孤児院に送ったという。苦しさから解放された喜びなのか、モムの死に顔はほほえむように優しかった。

2 Moum

In August 2002, one woman was in the dim ward, and she was feeding rice gruel to her daughter.

　Moum was 28 years old. She had wasted away just like an old woman. She rolled up her shirt, which was soaked with sweat. Her ribs stood out, as she showed her body of bones and skin. I was at a loss for words.

　"My body became thin like this. My body flushes all the time as though I am on fire inside. I wonder if I will dry up like ashes."

　I was worried whether I should take pictures. I put down my camera bag from my shoulder, and I turned an eye to the scene outside the window, when she said, "Look, take my picture." I took a camera, and peeped into the finder. There I saw the figure of a thin woman who had lost her vitality. In a small voice she sighed, "I want to escape from this pain as soon as possible"

　Exactly one month from that moment, death came to Moum. Several days before her death, she sent her daughter to the orphanage alone. Moum's face had a slight smile when she died. Maybe she felt some small joy because she was liberated from pain.

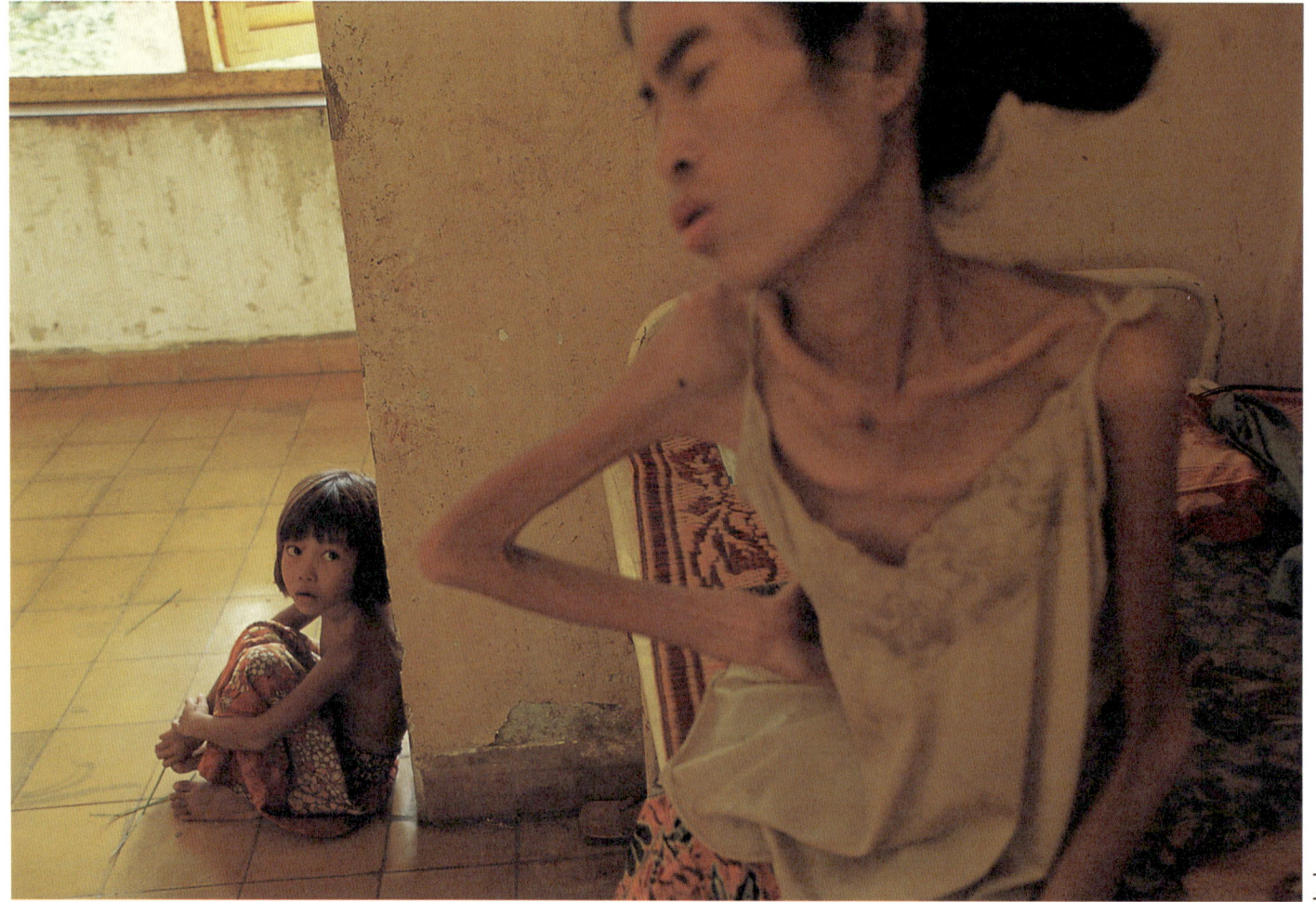

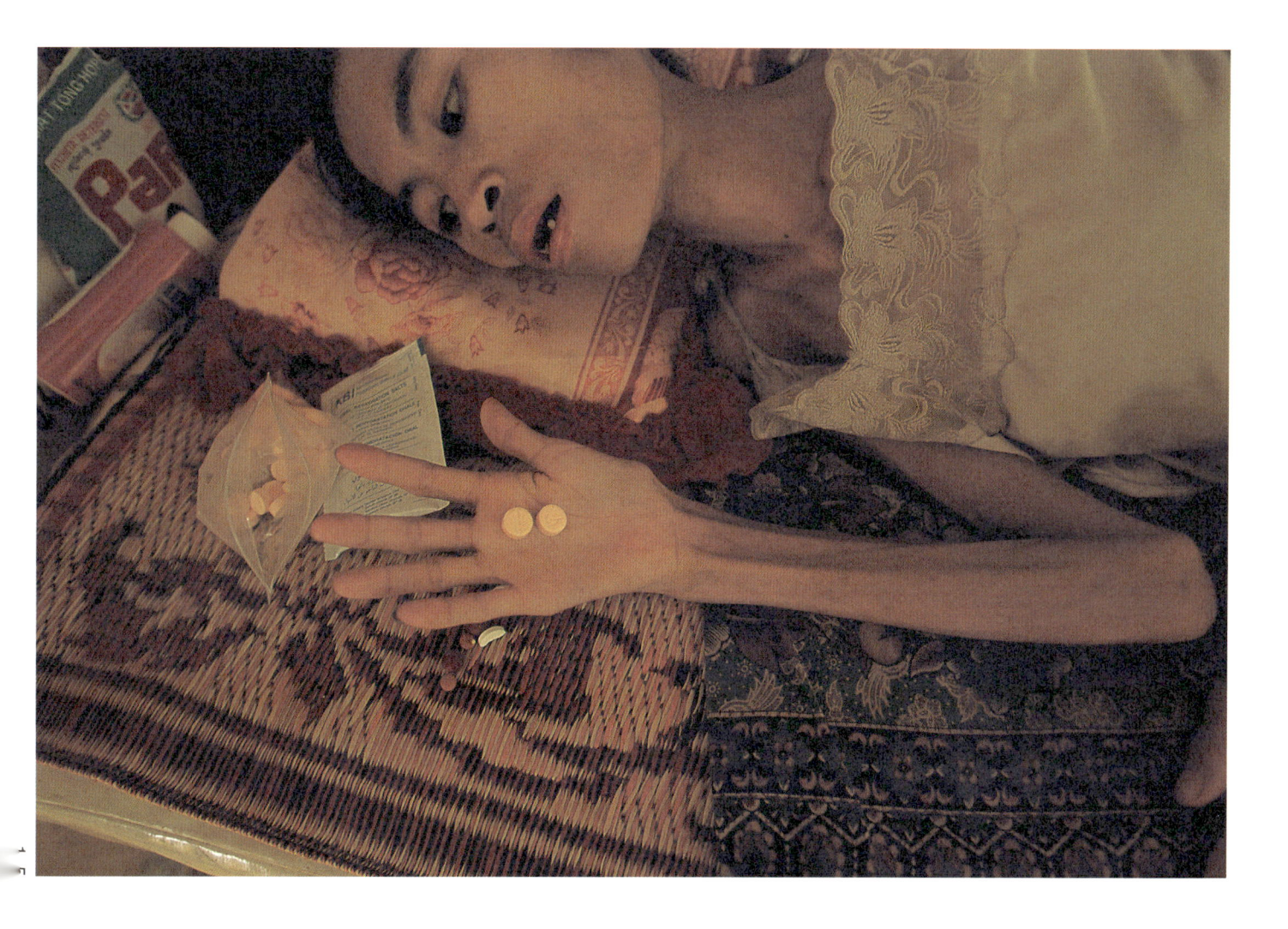

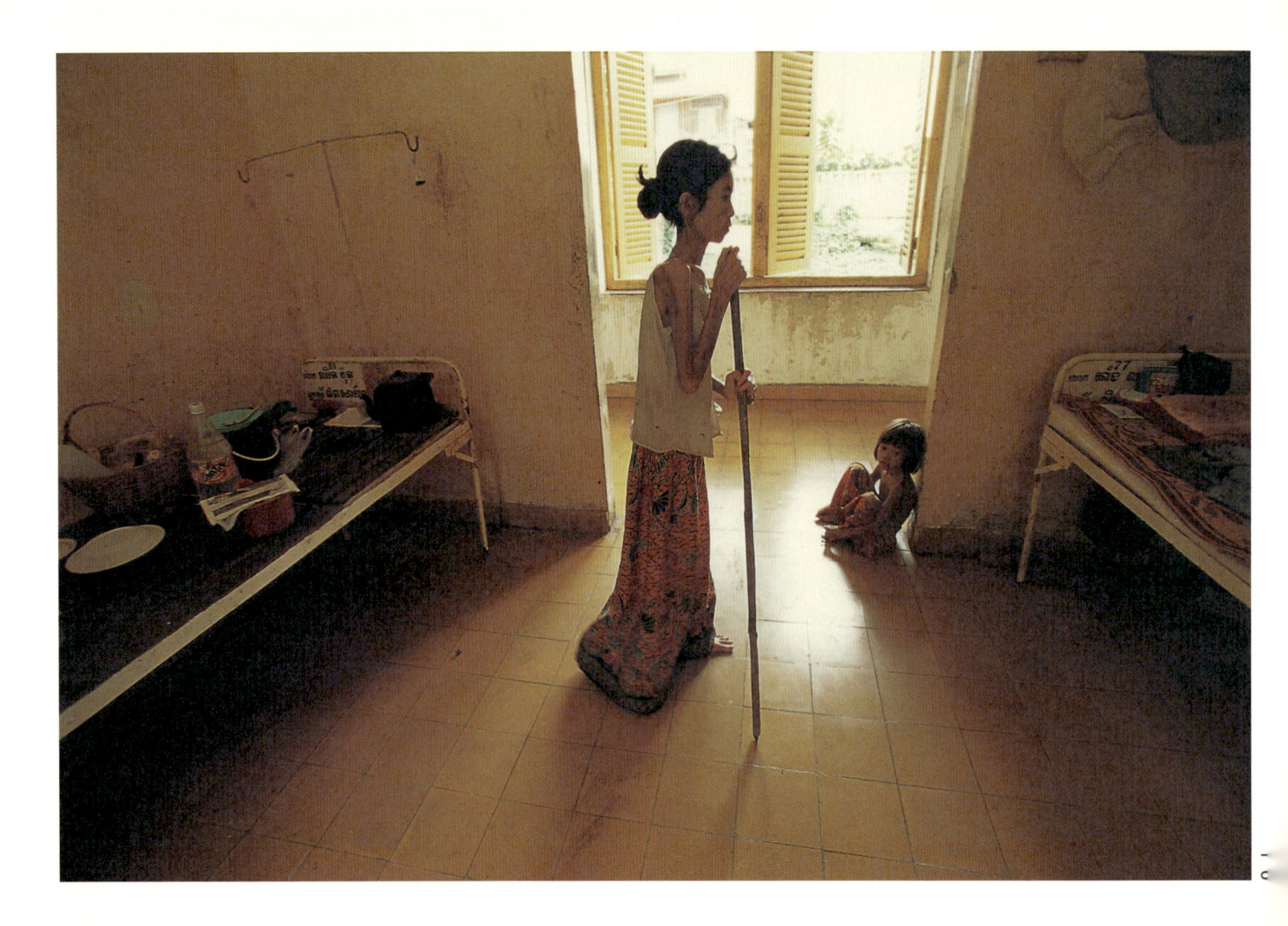

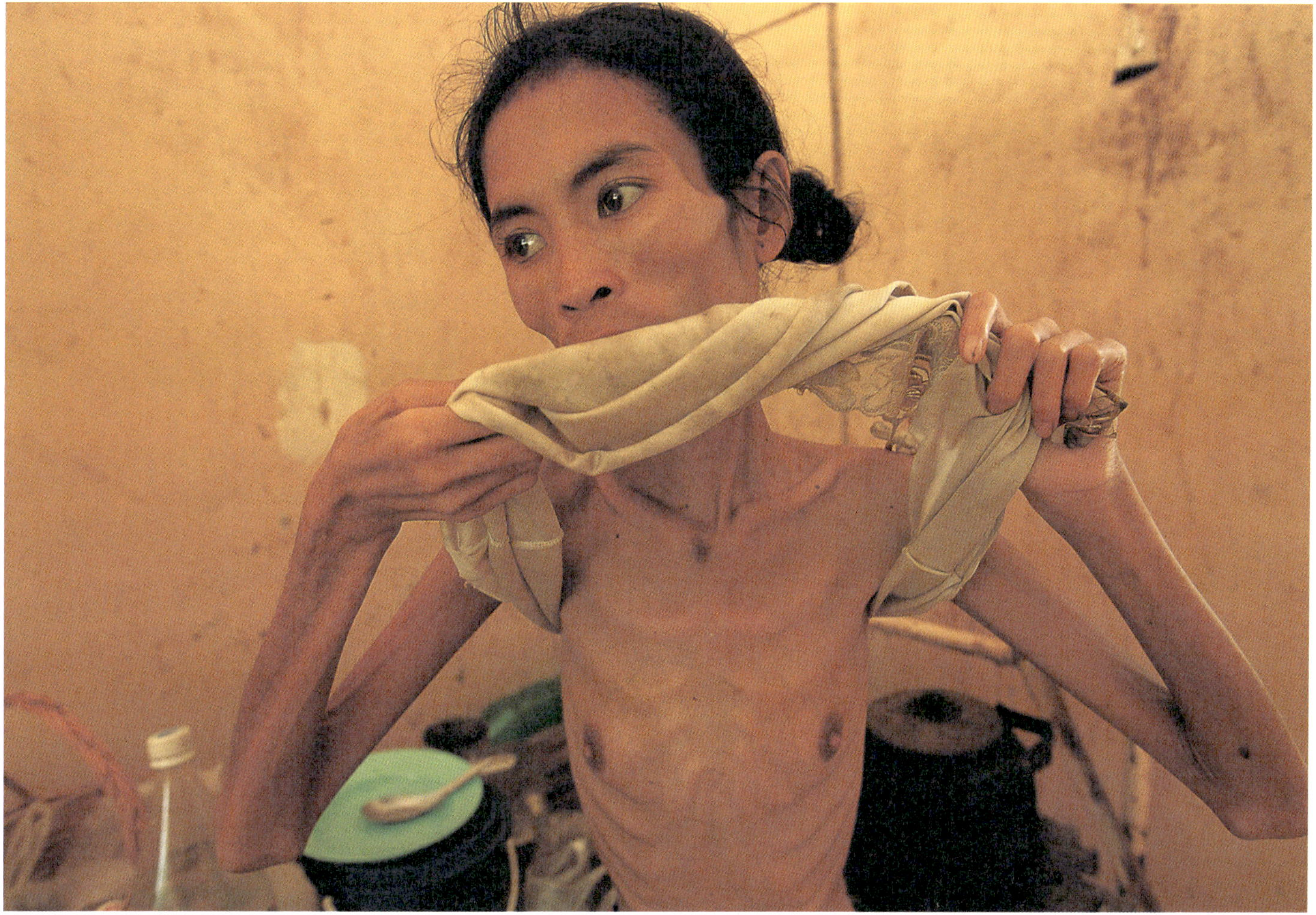

3　ソフィア

　2002年7月。ソフィアは1日中ベッドに横になって、いつも天井を眺めて、ただじっと時が流れるのを待っていた。

　27年前、彼女はベトナム国境沿いのスワイリエン州で生まれた。実家は貧しく、金に困った母親は16歳のソフィアを人買いに売ってしまった。彼女はタイの首都バンコクへ送られた。

　「時々男たちに白い液体を腕に打たれました。ウサギ小屋のような小屋で仲間と雑魚寝をし、朝から晩まで客をとらされました」

　体に異変が起きたのは1999年。病院で検査を受けると「エイズ」と診断された。組織の男たちに告げると、「二度と戻ってくるな」と言われ、あっけなく放り出された。ソフィアはそのまま夜行バスに乗り、カンボジア国境の町まで着いた。

　「髪の毛が抜け、黄疸が顔にも出ていました。体が醜くて、ずっと毛布で体を覆っていました」

　それからソフィアは日に日に衰弱した。起き上がることもできなくなったある日、暗い病室で彼女はひとりぼっちで死を迎えた。

3 Sophea

In July 2002, Sophea was in bed all day long, looking at the ceiling, waiting for the time to pass.

　She was born 27 years before in Svay Rieng province along the Vietnamese border. When Sophea was 16, her mother sold her to a child trafficker because the mother was pressed for money. The trafficker sent Sophea to the Thai capital, Bangkok.

　"Sometimes men injected white liquid (drugs) in my arm. I slept with many others in a hut like a rabbit hutch and I had to take 'guests' from the morning until the evening."

　It was 1999 when Sophea became sick with many illnesses all at once. She was diagnosed as HIV positive after a hospital examination. She told the men in her brothel that she had AIDS and they threw her out, saying, "Do not come back here again." Suddenly freed from her captors, she immediately caught a night bus for the Cambodian border.

　After her return, she says, "My hair came out, and jaundice appeared in my face as well. As my body became ugly, I covered myself with a blanket all the time."

　Sophea became weaker day by day. One day she couldn't get up any more, and she died alone in a dim room in the epidemic ward.

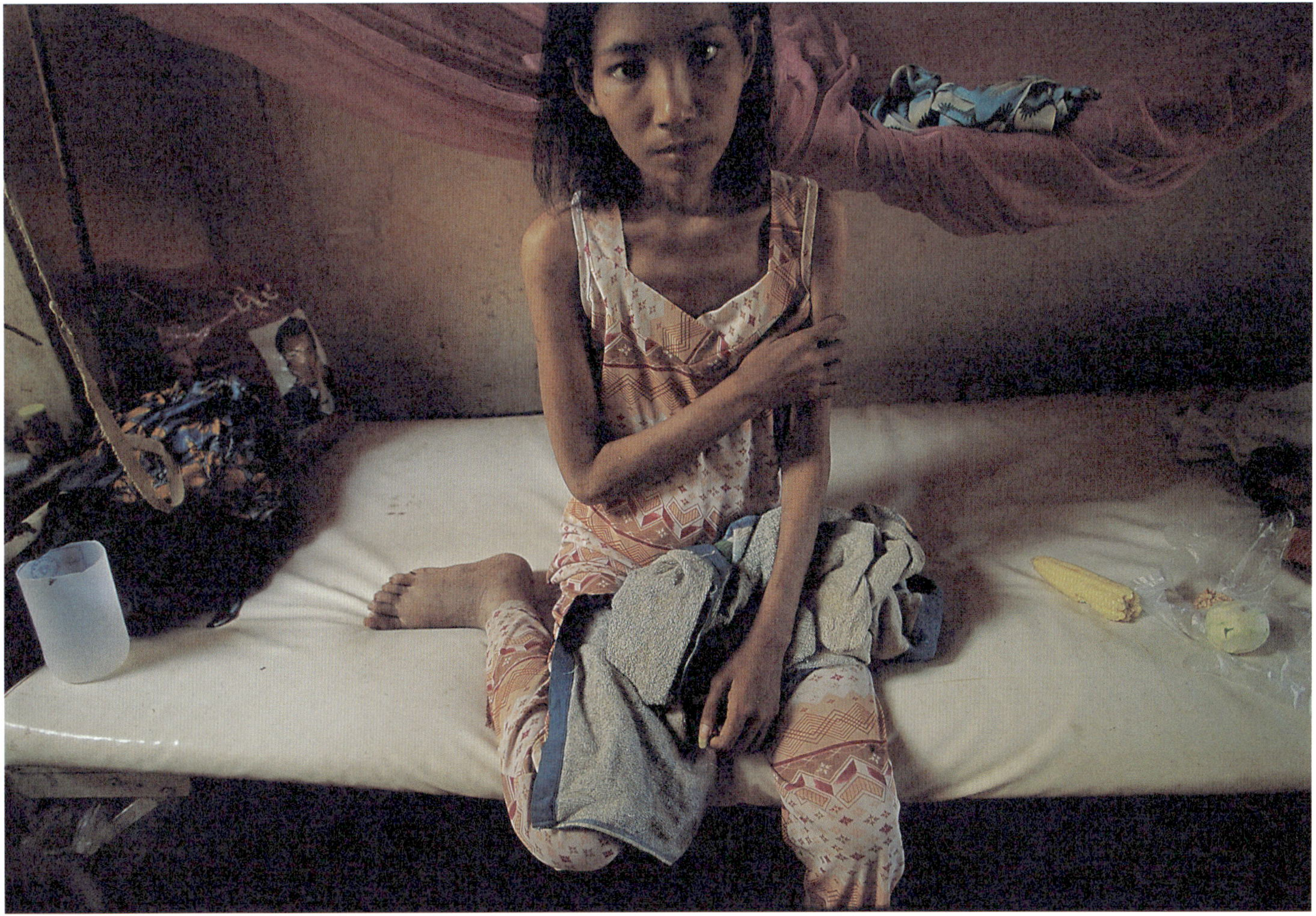

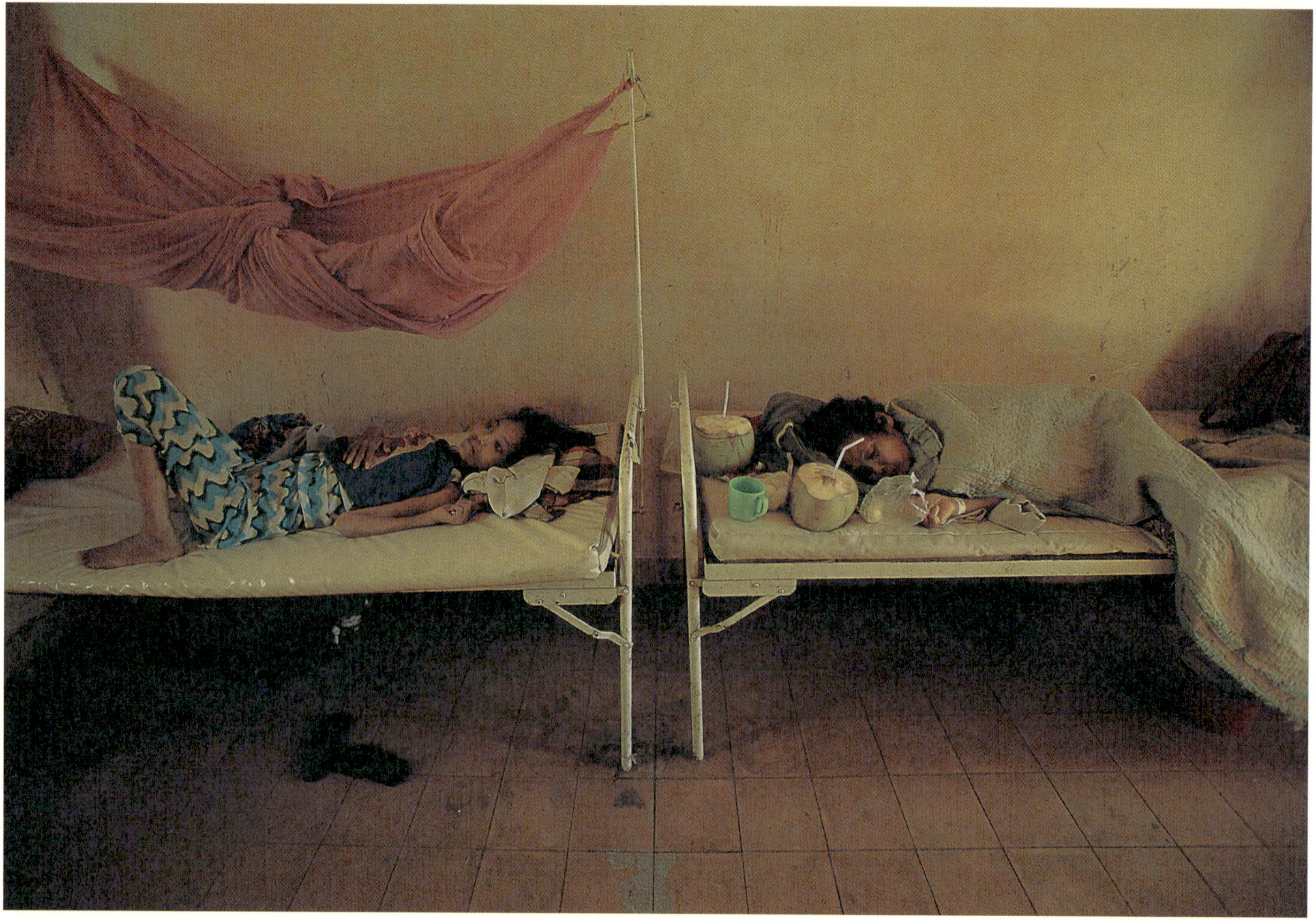

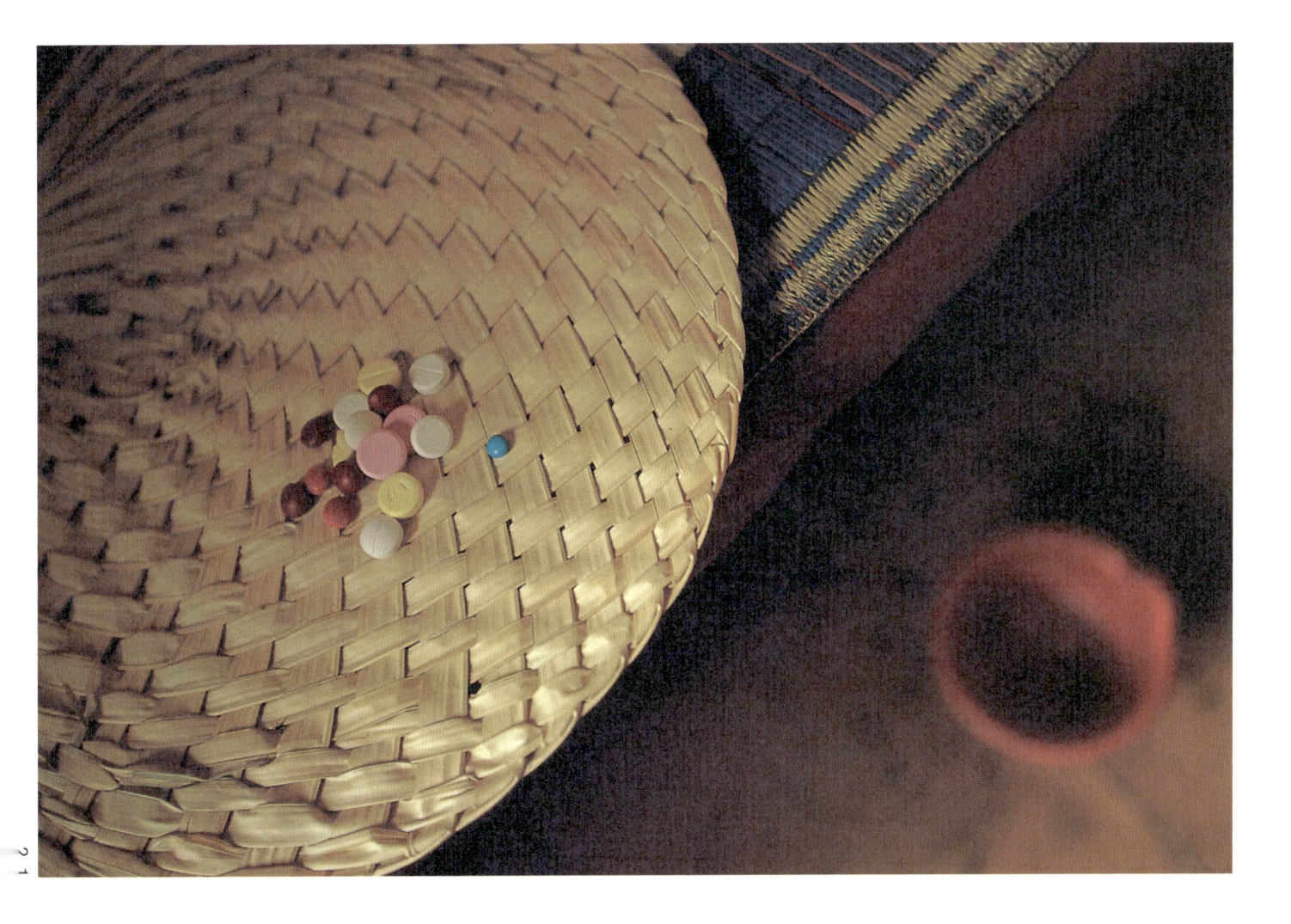

4 リム

　2002年6月。「そろそろ退院して故郷に帰りなさいと、お医者さんに言われました。もう私は駄目なのかしら」

　リムは老婆のように杖をついて歩く。「疲れた」と言って、何度も床に座り込んだ。

　「夫は私の目の前で、苦しみながら死にました」

　それだけ言うと、彼女は黙ってうつむいた。夫は2年ほど前、彼女にみとられながら、故郷シエムリアップの村で死んだ。エイズだった。夫は酒に酔うと女遊びをしていたので、それがエイズに感染した原因だったのだろう、と彼女は言った。そしてリムは、夫からエイズを感染させられた。

　1969年にシエムリアップ州で生まれたリムは、20歳の時に夫と結婚した。3人の子供がいるが、今は故郷で暮らす祖母が面倒をみている。

　「子供たちのことが心配です。私が死んだら、子供たちはどうなるのかしら。もし私が死んだら、残された子供たちを孤児院に入れてください」

　リムはそう言って、薄暗い病室の中で涙を流した。

　退院する日の朝、リムは病室で荷物をまとめていた。死が近づいていたことは、彼女自身が一番よく知っていたのだろう。死ぬ前にもう一度子供たちに会いたいと彼女は言っていた。最後に願いは叶った。リムが故郷の村に帰った後の消息はわからない。

4 Lim

In July 2002, I met a woman named Lim. She walked with a stick like an old woman. "The doctor told me that I can leave the hospital soon and go back home, but I wonder if I may die soon."

Lim sometimes said, "I get tired," and she sat down on the floor often.

"My husband suffered and died in front of me."

After she said these words, she bowed her head and became silent. Her husband died in their village in Siem Reap province about two years before, after being nursed by her. He had AIDS. He became infected with AIDS after sleeping with other women when he was drunk. And so, Lim was infected with AIDS by her husband.

Lim was born in 1969 in Siem Reap province and married when she was 20 years old. She has three children, and the children's grandmother now takes care of them in their home town. "I am worried about the children. If I die, what will happen to them? If I die, please take my children to an orphanage." she said to me, and then she shed tears in the dim room.

One morning, Lim collected her baggage and prepared to leave the hospital. She knew well that death was approaching. Before dying, she hoped to meet her children again. Though it was sad, her last wish was realized so close to the end. There was no news from her after she went back to her village.

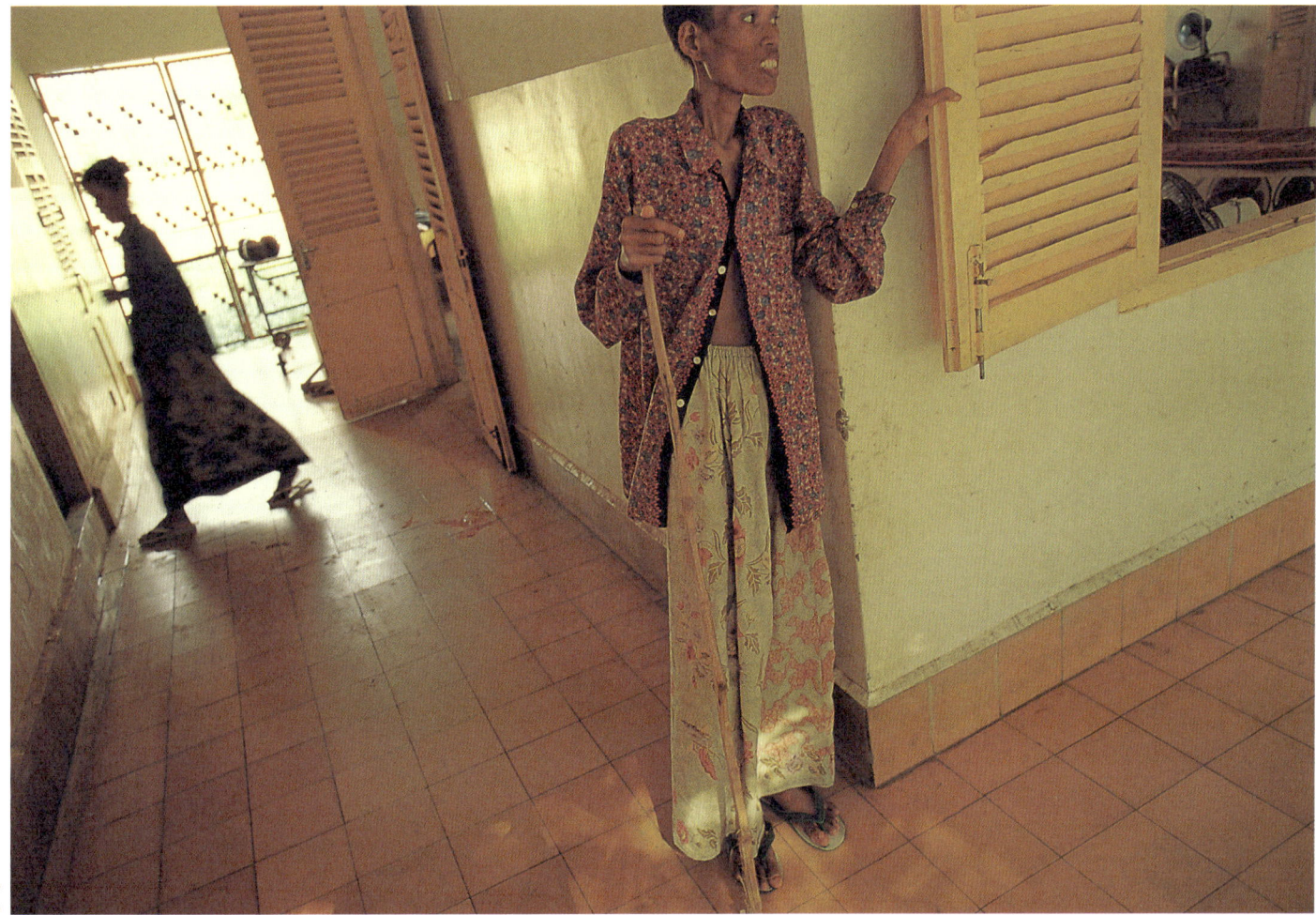

24

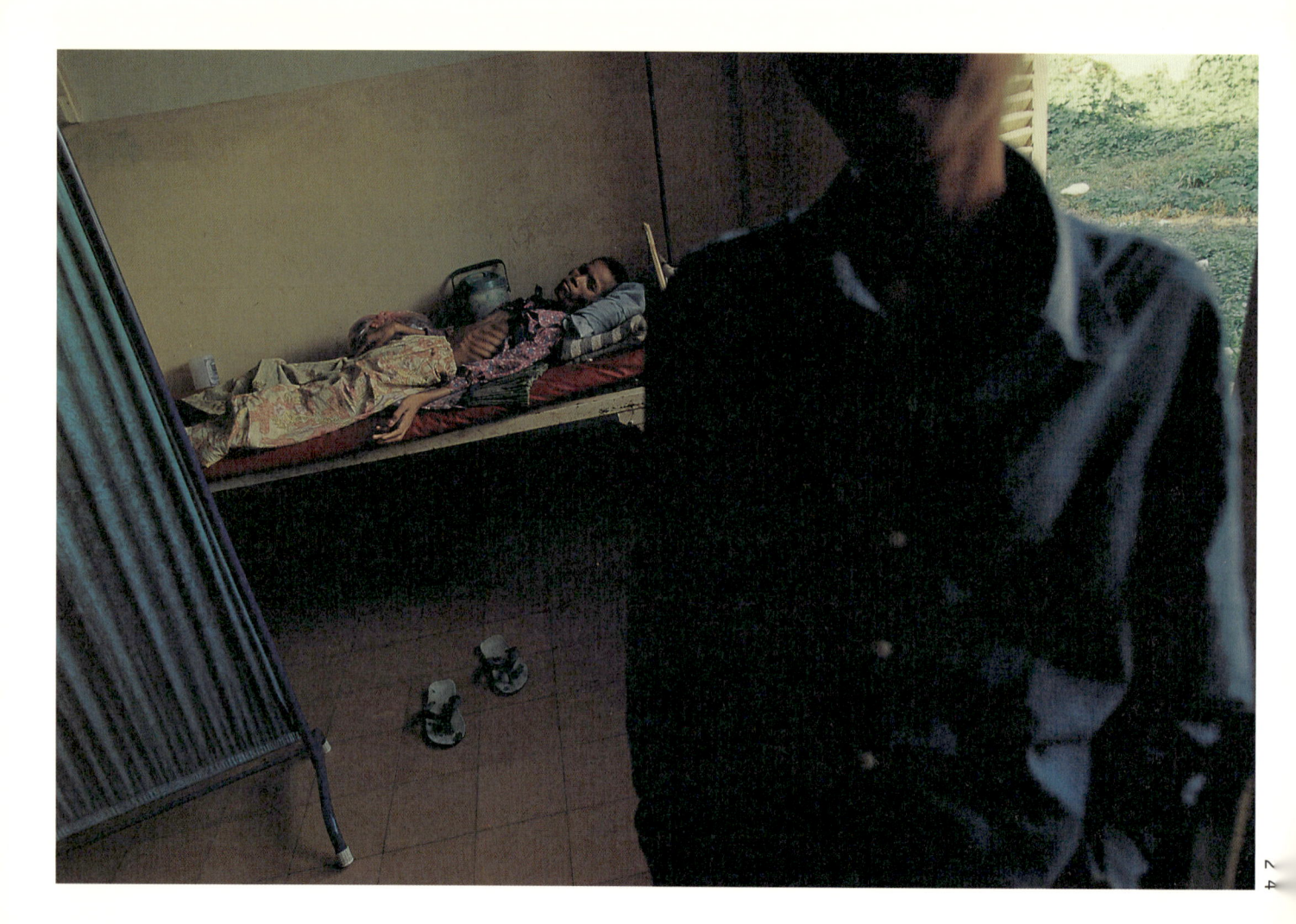

5 イン

　2002年6月。インは既に、風が吹けば倒れそうなくらい衰弱していた。横にいる妻はまだ若く22歳だという。彼は10歳年上で、4年前に結婚した。隣の空いたベッドの下に、小さな赤ん坊がハンモックの中で眠っていた。「結婚して2年目でやっと子供に恵まれた。子供はかわいいよ。あと3人は欲しい」

　バッタンバン州のスナン地区で生まれたインは、16歳の時に政府軍に入隊した。内戦後に政府軍が解体され、インは故郷の村に戻る。小さな土地を買い、家族と幸せに暮らしていた時、エイズを発症した。前線で負傷して治療を受けた時に、注射針を使い回ししていたためにエイズに感染したのだろうと彼は言った。

　「政府は酷いよ。戦争が終わって、俺たちをゴミのように捨てた。今俺がエイズになっても助けてもくれない」

　1週間後、妻は子供を連れて故郷に帰っていった。

　「お金が底をついた」1人残されたインが言う。家族のことを想っているのか、妻がお守り代わりに残していったという髪飾りをじっと見つめていた。

　2ヵ月後僕がまた病院に来た時、彼の姿はなかった。病状が悪化し、「死ぬ時は家で死にたい」と言い残して、インは故郷に帰ったという。

5　Ing

In July 2002, Ing was already weak and he seemed ready to fall down in the wind. His wife sitting next to him was still young; she said she was 22 years old. Ing was 10 years older than she, and they were married 4 years earlier. A little baby slept in a vacant bed under a hammock.

"After we got married, we were finally blessed with a child in our second year," said Ing. "A child is cute. We want to have at least three more."

Ing was born in Sunan district in Battambang province and joined the government army when he was 16 years old. After the civil war ended, government forces were dismantled and Ing returned to his village. Then, when he bought a little land and was living happily with his family, he found out that he had AIDS.

He said that he may have been infected with AIDS while a soldier, as they often shared needles for injections when they were injured in battle. "The government is cruel. We were left like trash because the war was finished. They don't help me even as I suffer from AIDS now."

One week after I met them, Ing's wife went back to their village with their child. "Money ran out already," said Ing, who was left alone. He might have been thinking of his family as he stared at the hair ornament his wife left with him as a memento. His wife seemed to be so sad when she left that Ing told her, "I will go back home when I get well." When I returned to the epidemic ward two months later Ing was not there. His condition became worse and he left for his village, telling the people at the hospital, "When I die, I want to die in my house."

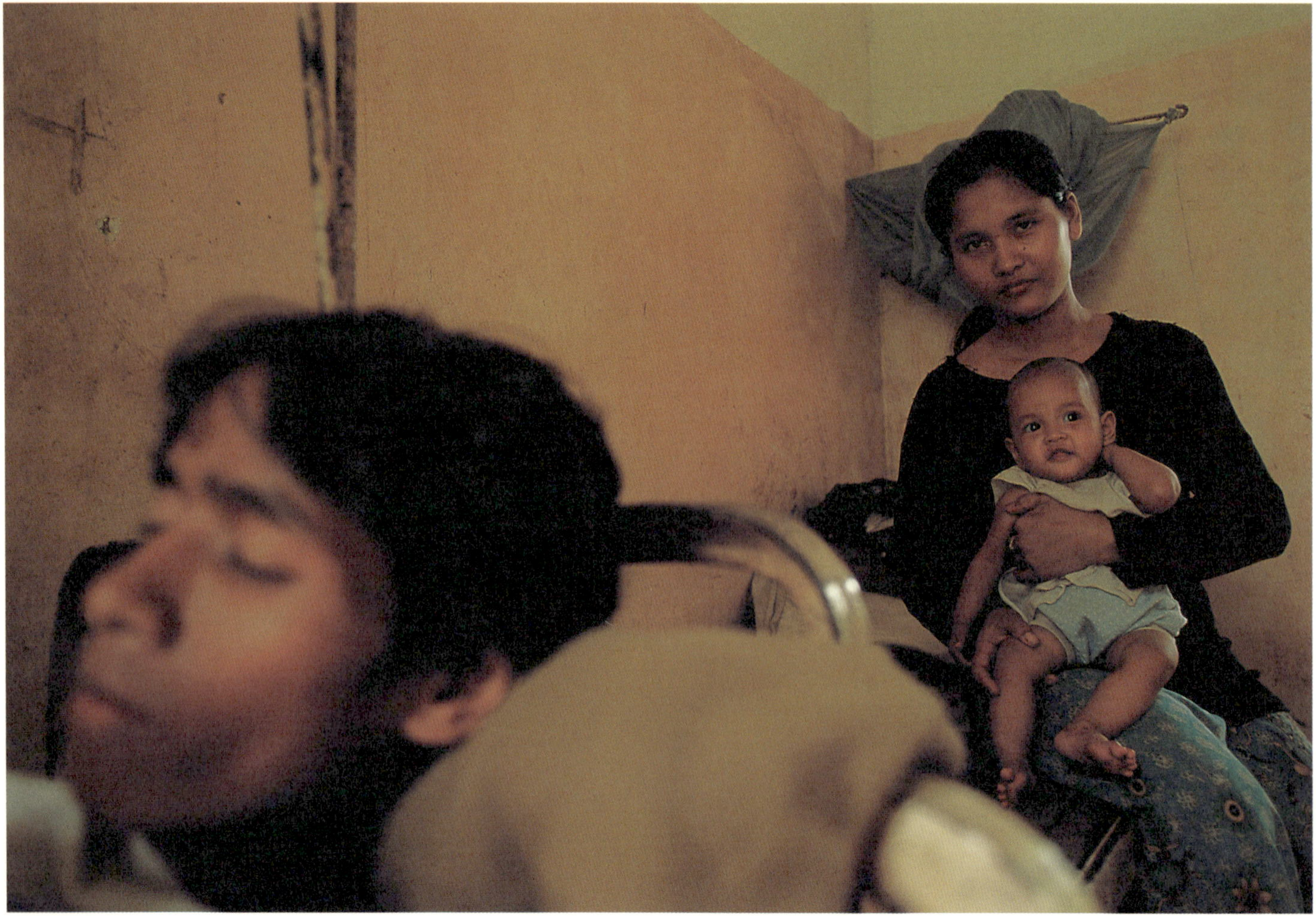

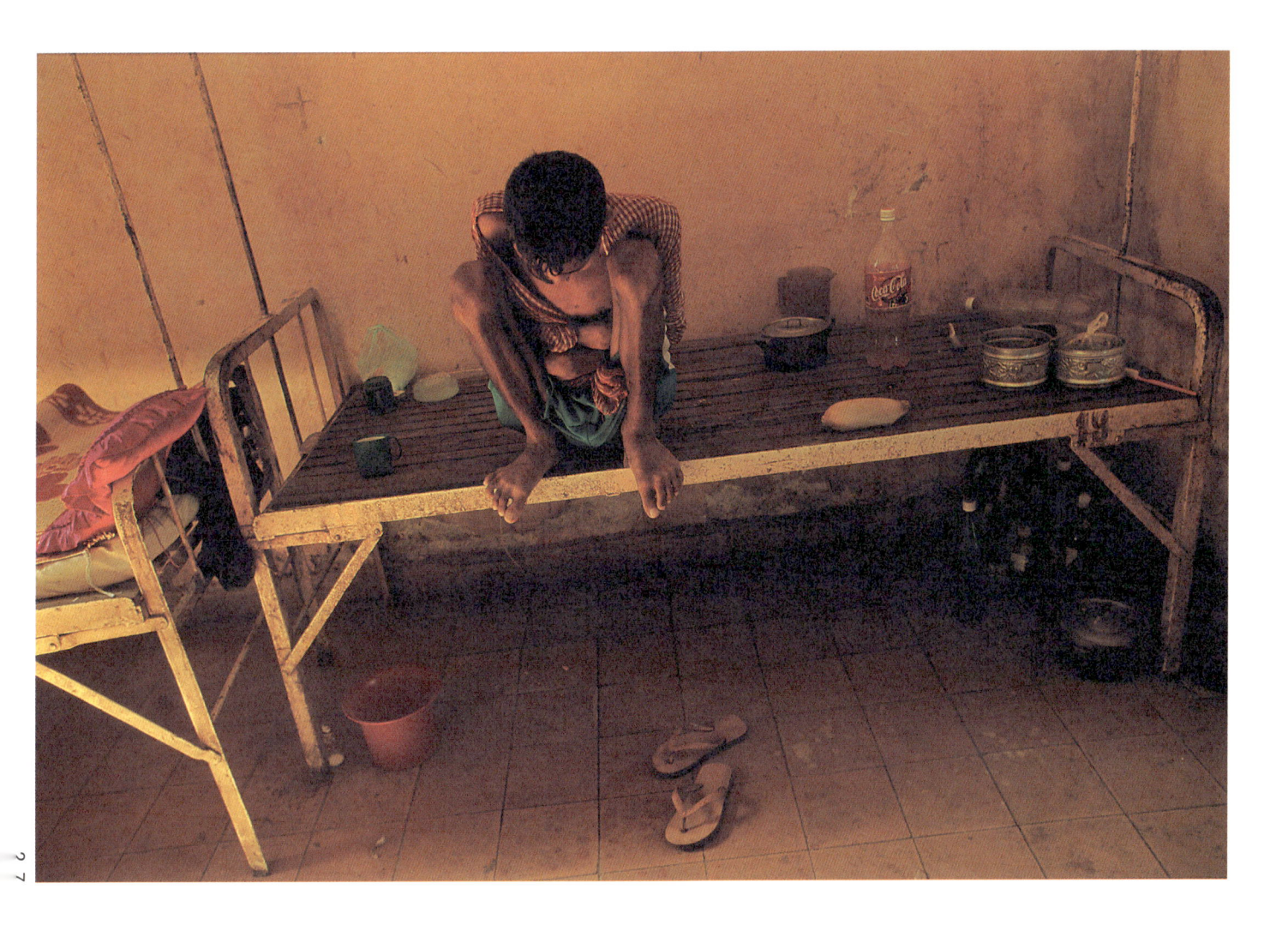

6　ラッタナー

　2002年5月。エイズ患者たちは1日に2000リエル（約40円）を援助団体から受け取る。ラッタナーはそのお金で甘いお菓子を買い、子供たちに与えていた。母と共に病院で暮らす長男のナリスは6歳、そして次男ダラは5歳になる。祖母がひとりシエムリアップにいるが、他に身寄りはないという。

　結核に罹っている彼女は、時折酷く咳き込み、苦しそうに唾を吐く。病棟では結核が原因で死に至るエイズ患者が最も多い。

　ラッタナーは1967年にアンコールワット付近の村で生まれた。13年間タイの難民キャンプで暮らしたあと、1991年に故郷に戻り、村の役場で働いていた夫と結婚した。その後、2人の子供に恵まれて幸せに暮らしていたが、1999年に夫がエイズを発症する。闘病は半年ほど続き、夫はこの世を去った。夫がエイズに感染した原因はわからないという。

　午後5時になり、病院の中庭から「カン、カン」と鐘の音が聞こえてきた。食事の時間だ。寝ていた子供たちが目を覚まし、お腹が空いたと泣き始める。

　「私は死にたくない。生きていたい。それもすべて、この子たちのためです」

　細く痩せた両腕でやさしく子供を抱きながら、ラッタナーはそう言った。

6　Rattana

Each day AIDS patients receive 2,000 Riel (0.50 US dollar) from Operations Enfants de Battambang (O.E.B), a local NGO (Non-Governmental Organization). Rattana bought sweets with that money, and she gave them to her children. Rattana suffers from tuberculosis, which is the actual cause of death for most AIDS patients in the epidemic ward. Sometimes Rattana has a bad coughing fit that leaves her exhausted and hacking multi-colored phlegm into a spittoon. Her eldest son, Narith, is six years old, and her second son, Dara, is five. They live in the hospital with their mother. Their only other relative is a grandmother in Siem Reap province.

　Rattana was born in a village near Angkor Wat temple in 1967. She lived in a Thai refugee camp for 13 years during the Vietnamese occupation, and returned to her village in 1991. There, she married a man who worked in the village government office. After that she was blessed with two children and a happy life. But in 1999 Rattana's husband got AIDS. Her husband fought the disease for half a year, but he died and left this world. She does not know how her husband was infected with HIV.

　It was 5 p.m., and a bell sounded like "Kan, Kan, Kan," from the courtyard in the hospital. It was dinner time. Sleeping children started to wake up and cry from hunger.

　"I don't want to die. I want to live. All of this for my children," Rattana said as she held a child gently with her thin, thin arms.

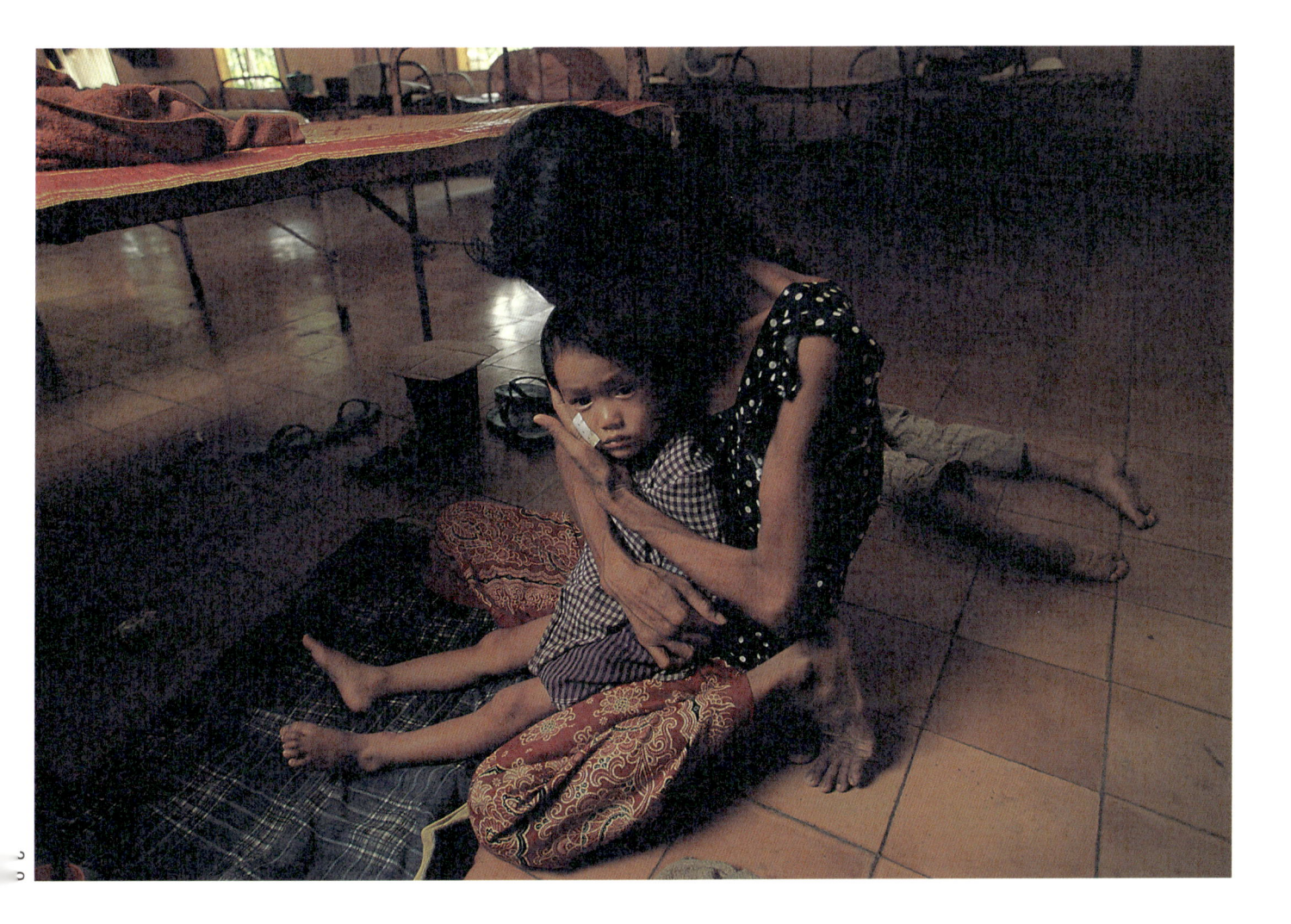

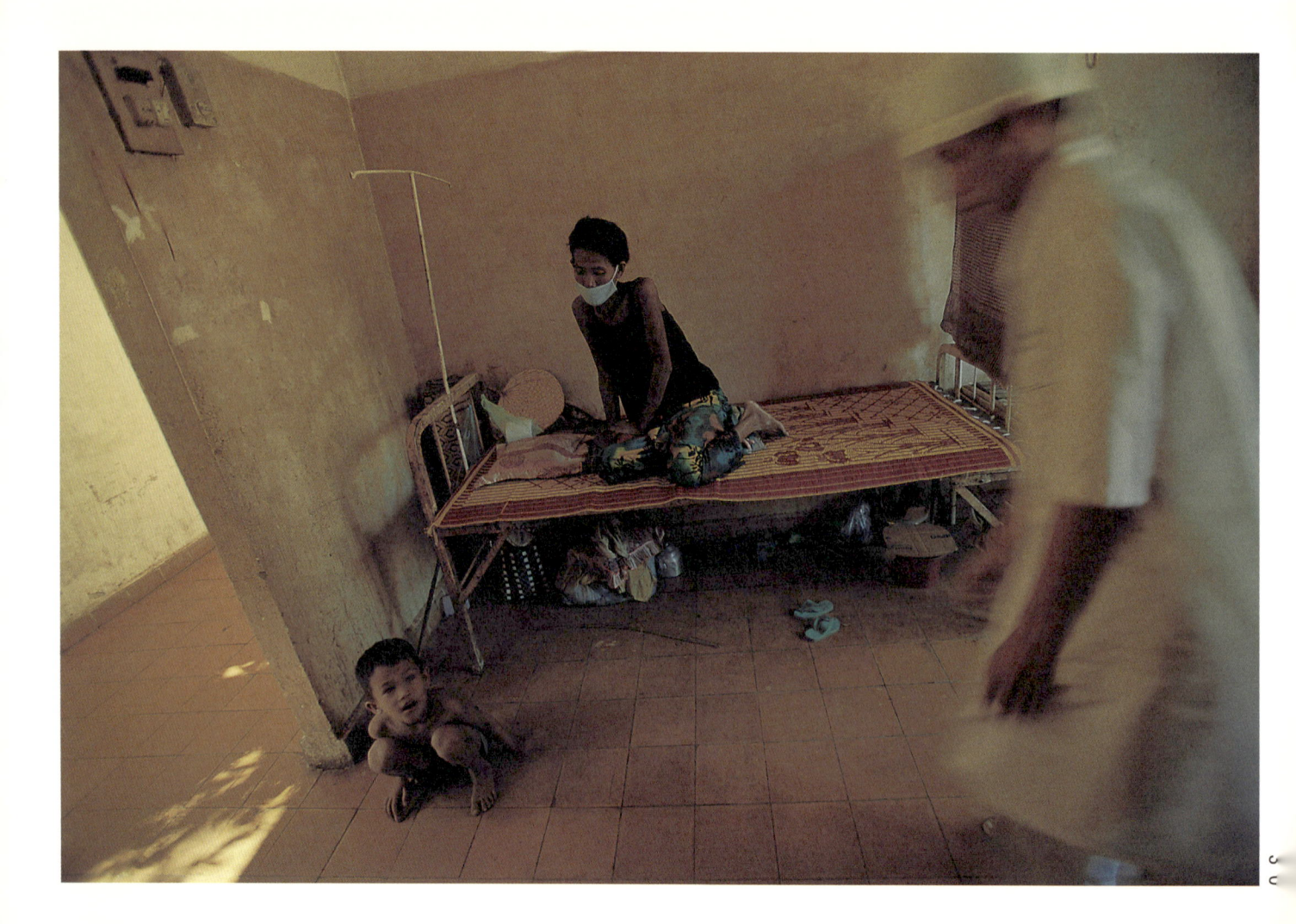

7 サオ

　2003月2月。リヤカーに乗せられて、1人の男性が感染病棟に運ばれてきた。苦しそうに顔を歪めながら、一緒にいる妻の手を握り締めている。サオという名で、子供が2人いる。1人は5歳くらい、もう1人はまだ生まれて間もないようだ。

　家族はタイ国境の町から、6時間以上かけて病院に着いた。車代は家族4人で20ドル以上かかったという。

　「手元にある残りのお金は、あとわずかしかない。どうしたらよいのか」

　妻が疲れ果てた表情で言う。

　末期症状で苦しむ夫をスセップ医師が診察する。注射を何本か打ち、看護師が血液を採った。痛みに耐えているサオの目から時折涙がこぼれ、妻がそっとぬぐってやった。

　「ああ、夫を助けてください。みなさん、お願いします」

　スセップ医師は妻に冷静になるように伝えた。看護師は絶望的な表情をする。苦しむ夫の横で、子供を抱えた妻はいつまでも涙を流していた。

7 Sao

In February 2003, one man arrived at the epidemic ward on a hand cart. He and his family came to the hospital from their village on the Thai border. They spent more than six hours and 20 US dollars - nearly all their money - to get here. The man rode on the hand cart for the last distance across the hospital grounds to the epidemic ward. It is the same cart the hospital uses to transport dead bodies. The husband's name is Sao and he has 2 children. One is about five years old; another one looks under six months.

　"We have only a few dollars left, what should we do now?" the wife asked, her expression exhausted.

　Sao grasped his face and held his wife's hand tightly.

　Doctor Sutthep examined Sao, who had the symptoms of a terminal condition. A few injections were given, and a nurse took his blood. Tears sometimes spilled from Sao's eyes as he bore the pain. His wife wiped her husband's tears gently.

　"Please, please help my husband. I am asking all of you," she pleaded.

　Doctor Sutthep said to her, "Please calm down." A nearby nurse had a hopeless look. As the husband suffered, his wife held their child next to him, shedding tears.

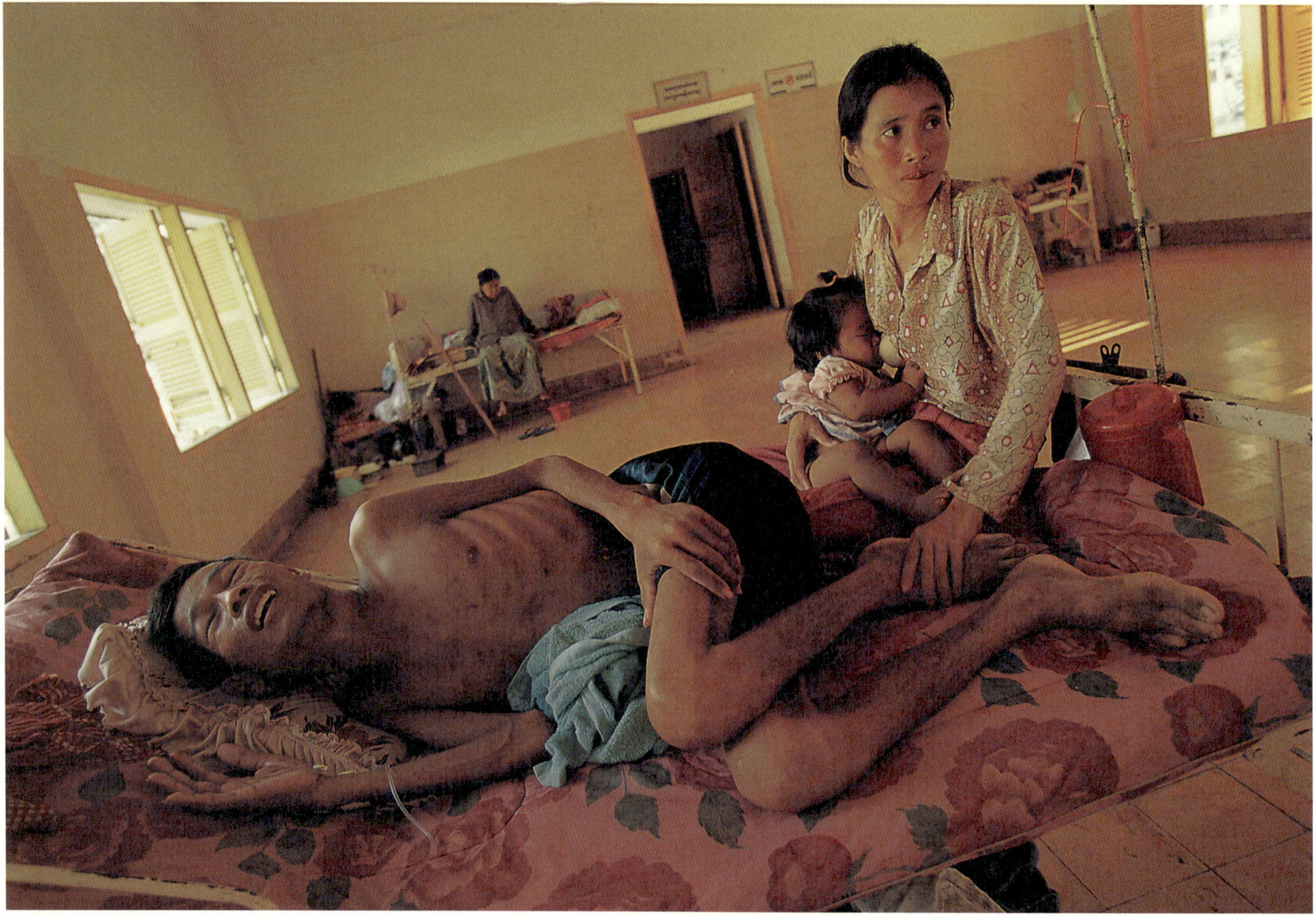

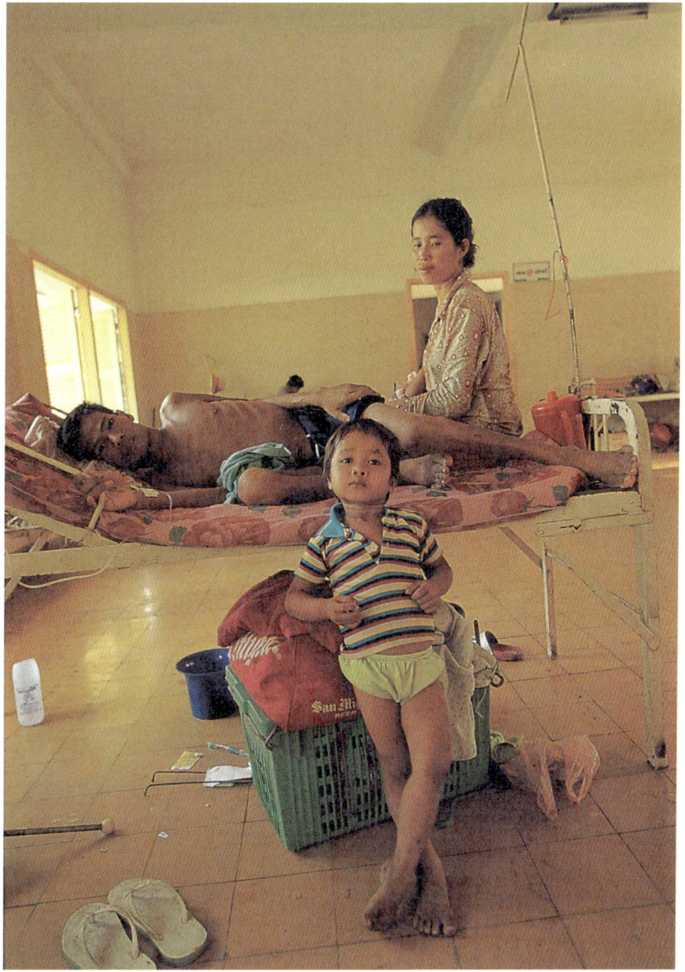

8 サビンとリン

　2003年2月。1組の姉妹が感染病棟にいた。姉のサビンは31歳、エイズを発症して1年が経っていた。8歳年下の妹のリンは、いつも姉を一生懸命看病していた。

　姉妹が病院に来たのは1ヵ月ほど前だった。

　「酷い頭痛が続き、病院で医師から血液検査をすすめられました。不安でした。2年前に別れた夫が今エイズで苦しんでいると聞いていたからです」

　検査の結果を見たサビンは絶望した。夫から感染したのは間違いなかった。

　父親は姉妹が幼い時、別の女性と家を出た。やさしかった母は十数年前に病死、頼りになった兄は94年に戦死してしまう。それ以来、姉妹は助け合いながら生きてきた。

　「姉の耐えている苦しさと比べると、看病など辛くありません。エイズに負けないでと、姉にいつも言っています」

　日中の強い日差しは、病室の中を砂漠のような暑さにする。高熱が続いて汗だくになった姉の体を、リンはやさしくタオルで拭いていた。

8 Savin and Lin

In February 2003, there was one pair of sisters in the epidemic ward. The older sister was Savin who was 31 years old. She already had AIDS for one year. Lin was eight years younger, and she always nursed Savin sincerely. The sisters came to the hospital about one month earlier.

"I divorced my husband two years ago and now I heard that he was suffering from AIDS," she continued. "It was difficult." But things became more difficult. "A severe headache lasted, and a doctor recommended blood tests in the hospital," Savin said. Then Savin saw the results of her blood tests, and she despaired. She was certain that she was infected by her husband.

When the sisters were little, their father left their home with another woman. Their mother was gentle, but died from an unknown sickness about 10 years ago. Their older brother was a reliable person, but was killed in battle in 1994. Since then, the sisters have helped each other.

"Nursing isn't severe if compared with the pain my older sister bears. I always tell my older sister, 'Don't give in to AIDS.'"

The strong sunlight in daytime heats the inside of the epidemic ward just like a desert. Savin was sweating from a high fever, and I watched Lin gently wipe her sister's body with a towel.

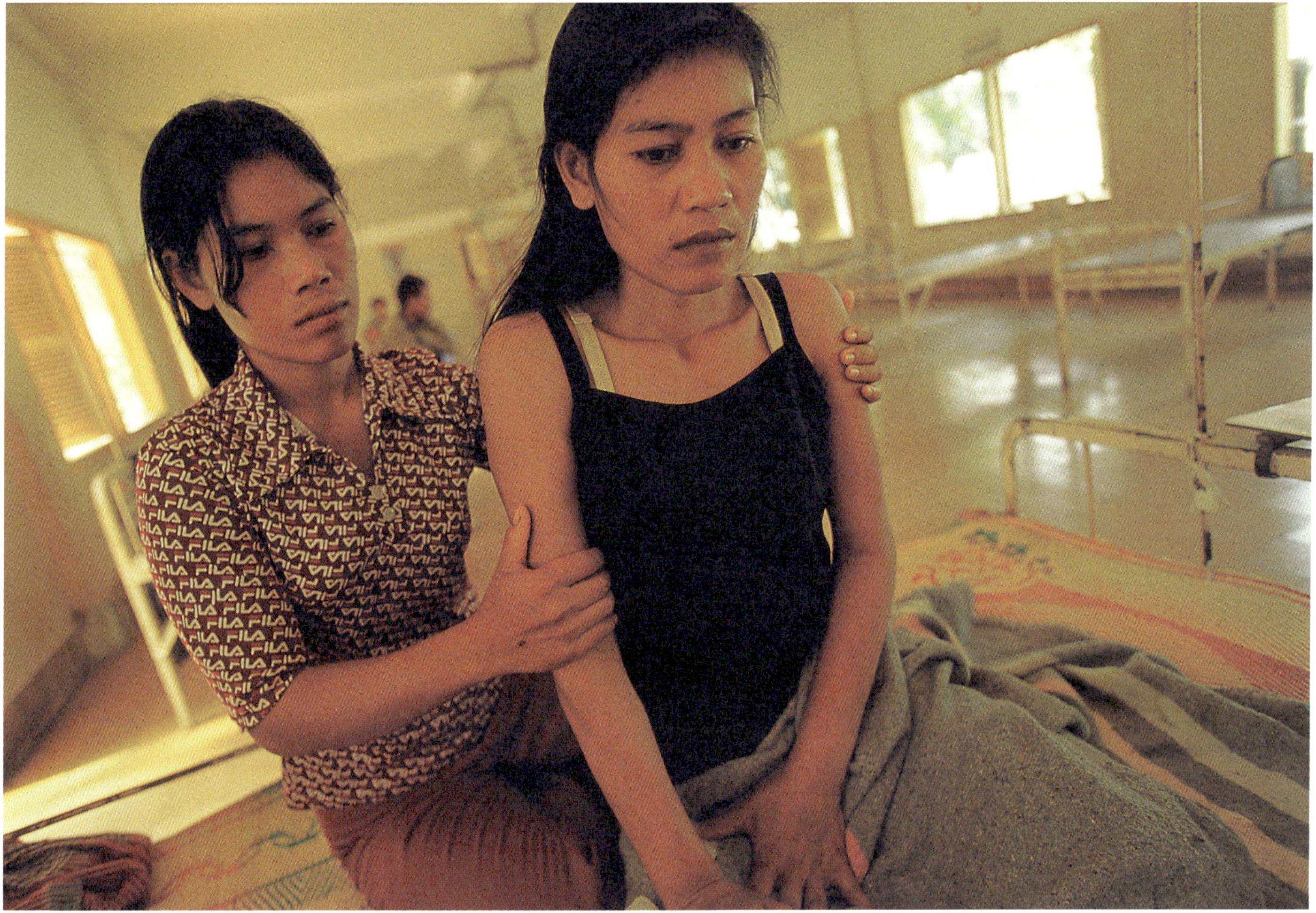

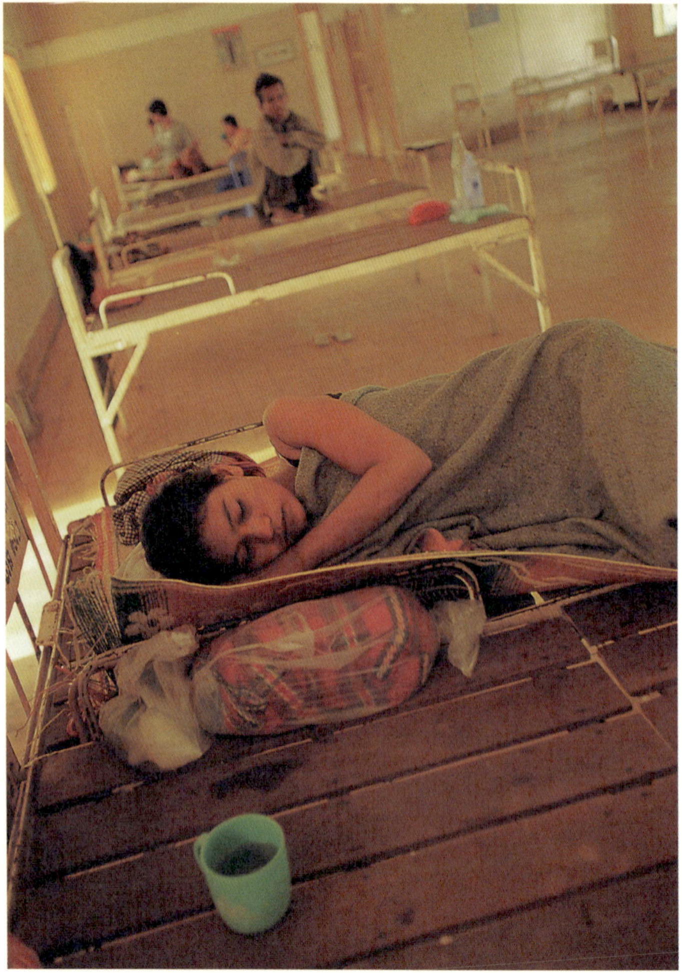

9 変わりゆく首都

　プノンペンの夜。ネオンが輝くディスコでは、ダンスミュージックが鼓膜が破れるくらいの大音量で流れ、若者たちは朝まで踊り明かす。

　野外ホールでのライブには、毎回、数百人の観客が集まる。眉を細く整え、スリムな体に流行のファッションで着飾ったアイドルたちがステージの上でヒップホップのリズムに合わせて踊っている。

　内戦後、都市では伝統的な価値観は失われ、権力と金が何より重要なものとなった。若者たちは無責任なセックスに走り、それがエイズの広がる原因となった。カンボジアは内戦で数百万人の国民を失った。そのため、現在、20歳以下が国民全体の54・8％を占めるという人口構成になっている。国連エイズ合同計画（UNAIDS）によると、カンボジア国内では毎日新たに20人がHIVに感染しているが、その感染者の半分が24歳以下だという。

　しかし、外国資本も入って街が活気づいているのも事実だ。プノンペンには内戦当時はなかった専門学校も増え、語学や技術を学ぶ場もできた。真新しいコンピューターの専門学校には、真剣な眼差しでパソコンに向かう若者たちの姿があった。彼らはカンボジアを再建できるのだろうか。

9 Phnom Penh Changes

　It is evening in Phnom Penh. The neon-sparkle discos open, the music flows out in huge waves and the young people dance until morning. Hundreds of people gather at an outdoor live music show. Idols put on their showy costumes and dance to the hip-hop rhythm on the stage. Their eyebrows are thin, and they dress up in slim body suits, the latest sexy fashion.

　After the civil war ended, the traditional values of the country were lost. Power and money have become two important symbols in the city. Cambodia lost several million people in the civil war, mostly adults. Because of that, today, 55% of Cambodians are under 20 years old. According to UNAIDS, about 20 people are infected with HIV in Cambodia every day. Half of those infected are under 24. Many have irresponsible sex and further spread the disease.

　But foreign capital comes in, too, and Phnom Penh is enlivened in another way. Vocational schools have sprung up across Phnom Penh, places to learn linguistics and technology. Good schools were uncommon during the civil war. In a new computer vocational school, I see young people facing their computers with serious looks. I wonder if they can rebuild Cambodia.

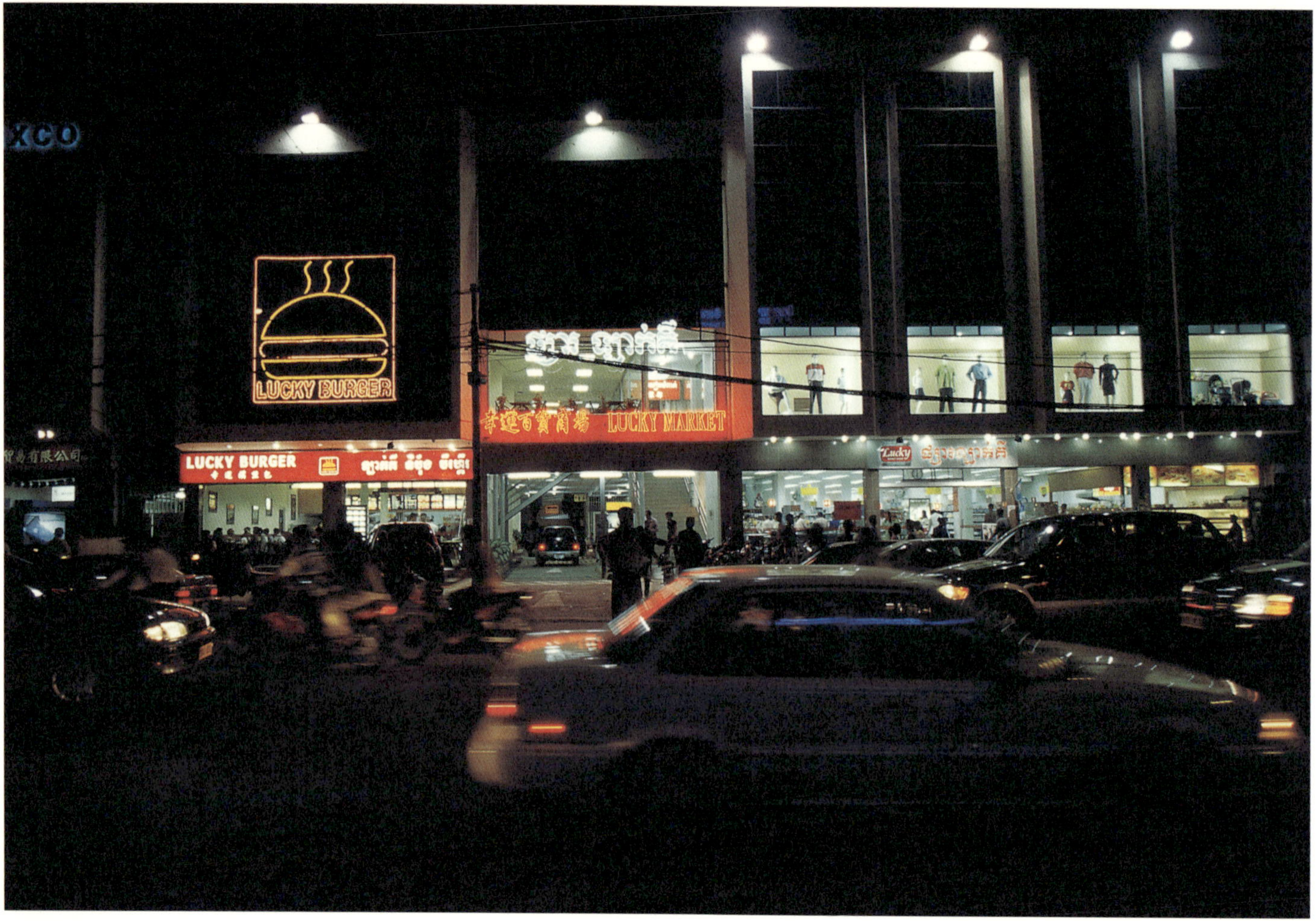
LUCKY BURGER
LUCKY BURGER
幸運百貨商場 LUCKY MARKET
Lucky

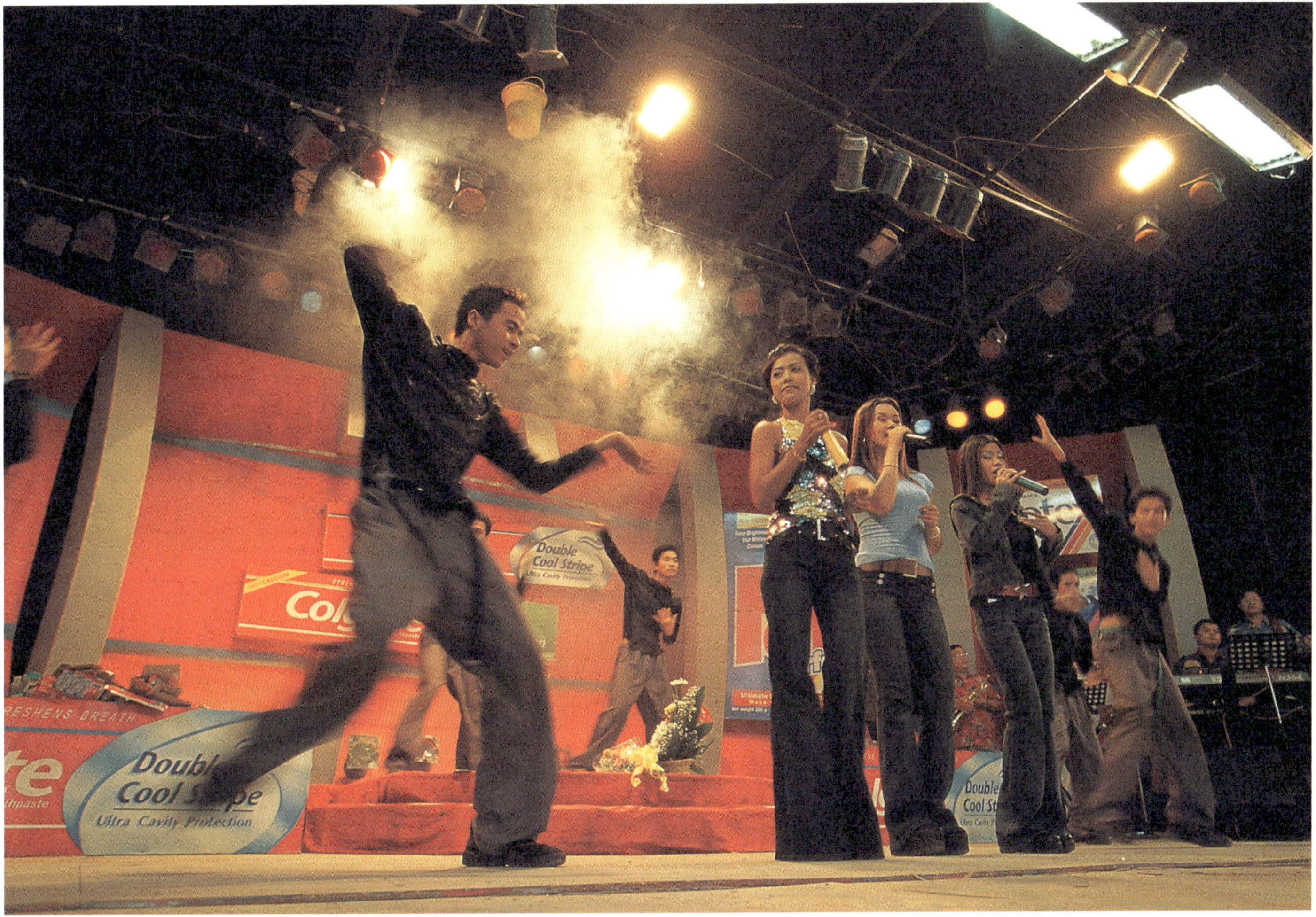
Double
Cool Stripe
Ultra Cavity Protection
RESHENS BREATH

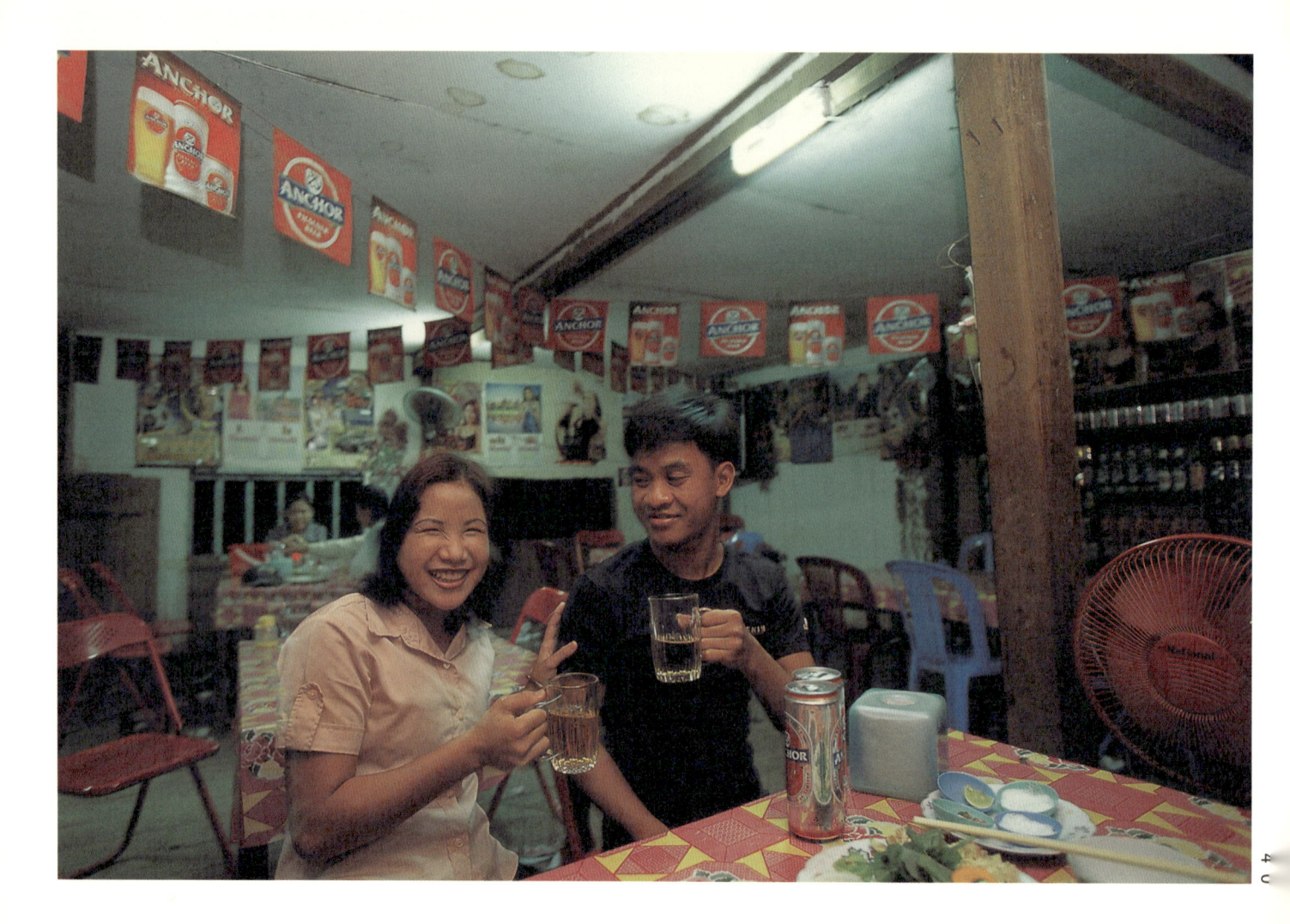

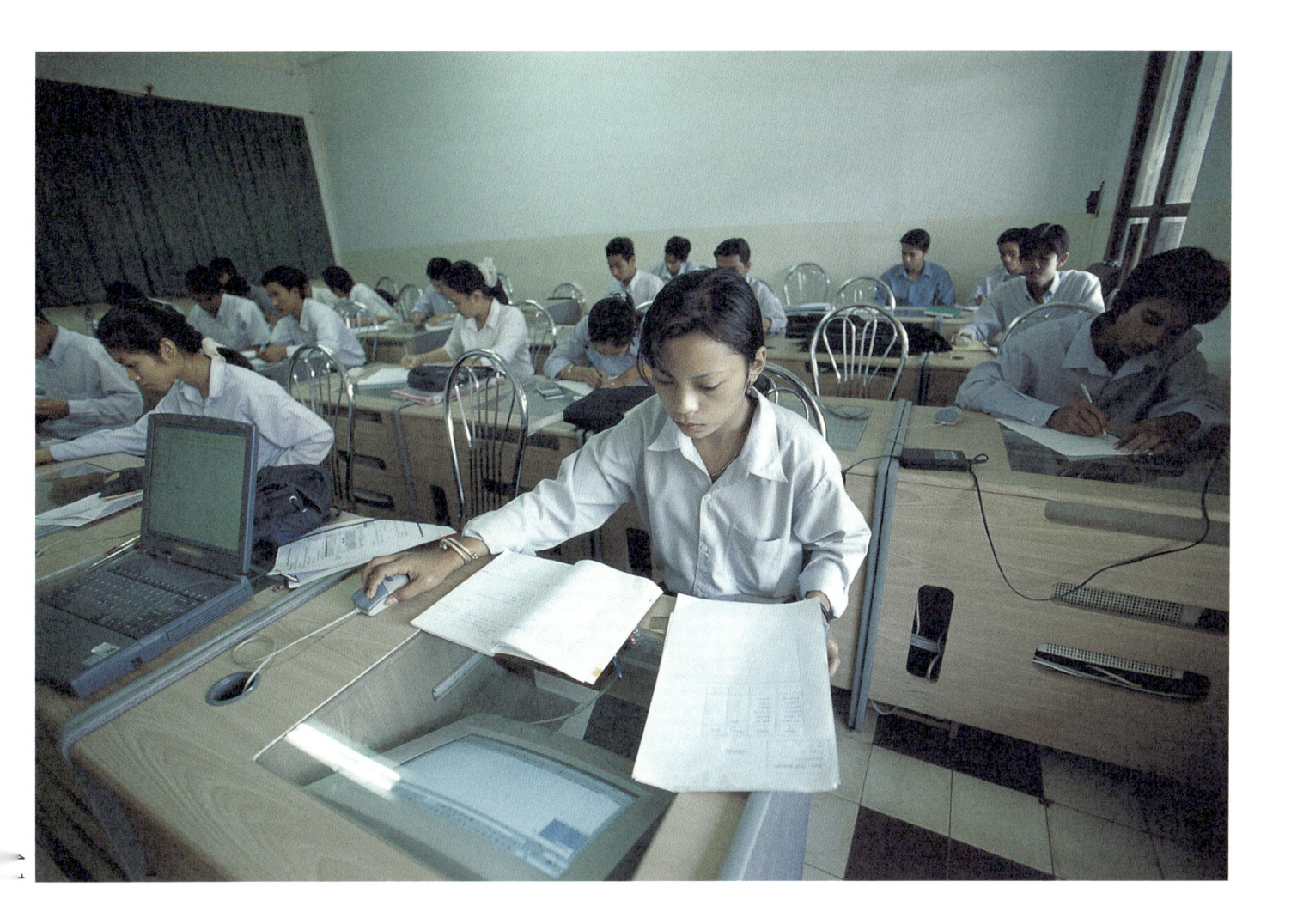

10 売られる子供たち

　2003年1月。タイとの国境の町ポイペトには1本の橋が架かっている。その橋脚の間に死んだように眠っている子供たちがいた。みな児童売買組織に売られた子供たちだ。

　朝日が昇る頃、汚れた川の水で子供たちは顔を洗った。全員が背中に衣類や雑貨を背負い、川を渡って藪の中に消える。一緒についていくと、細い獣道があり、しばらく行くとタイ側に入った。子供たちは検問を避けて荷物を運ぶ。違法な行為だが、ポイペト一帯を取り仕切る密売組織は、タイの官憲と手を組んでいるので平気だ。

　子供たちを支援している援助団体「フレンズ」のエングさんが言った。

　「一度、橋の下に行き、子供たちの話を聞きました。しかしすぐ男たちが来て、私を『今度来たら殺す』と脅しました。ここポイペトには巨大な闇組織が裏にあり、私たちにも助けることができないのです」

　虐待を受けながら、子供たちは1日中働いている。現在、カンボジアから国境を越えて売られる子供たちの数は、1ヵ月400人から800人いると言われている。

10 Trafficked Children

In January 2003, one bridge spans the gap between Poi Pet town and Thailand. There are children sleeping between the bridge pillars, dying. The children were sold into this life by child traffickers.

　When the morning sun rises, the children wash their faces with dirty water from the river below. Then they shoulder clothes and miscellaneous goods in bundles on their small backs and cross the river, disappearing into the bushes on the far side of the river, into Thailand. I follow them for a short distance, along thin animal trails through the brush. Later, they arrive at a market near the border. They are smuggling clothes and other goods into Thailand. Though it is illegal, there is no problem because the traffickers who work in Poi Pet town work with the Thai authorities. The children avoid inspection while carrying the bundles.

　Mr. Eng works with Friends, an NGO supporting children. He said, "I went under the bridge once, and listened to the children's stories. But men quickly came after me, and I was threatened: 'If you come again, we will kill you.'"

　Eng said that there are powerful forces behind the child-trafficking industry. "In Poi Pet, there is a huge darkness behind, so we can't help the children," he said.

　Meanwhile, the children are treated cruelly, and they work all day long. Between 400 and 800 children are trafficked across the border and sold each month.

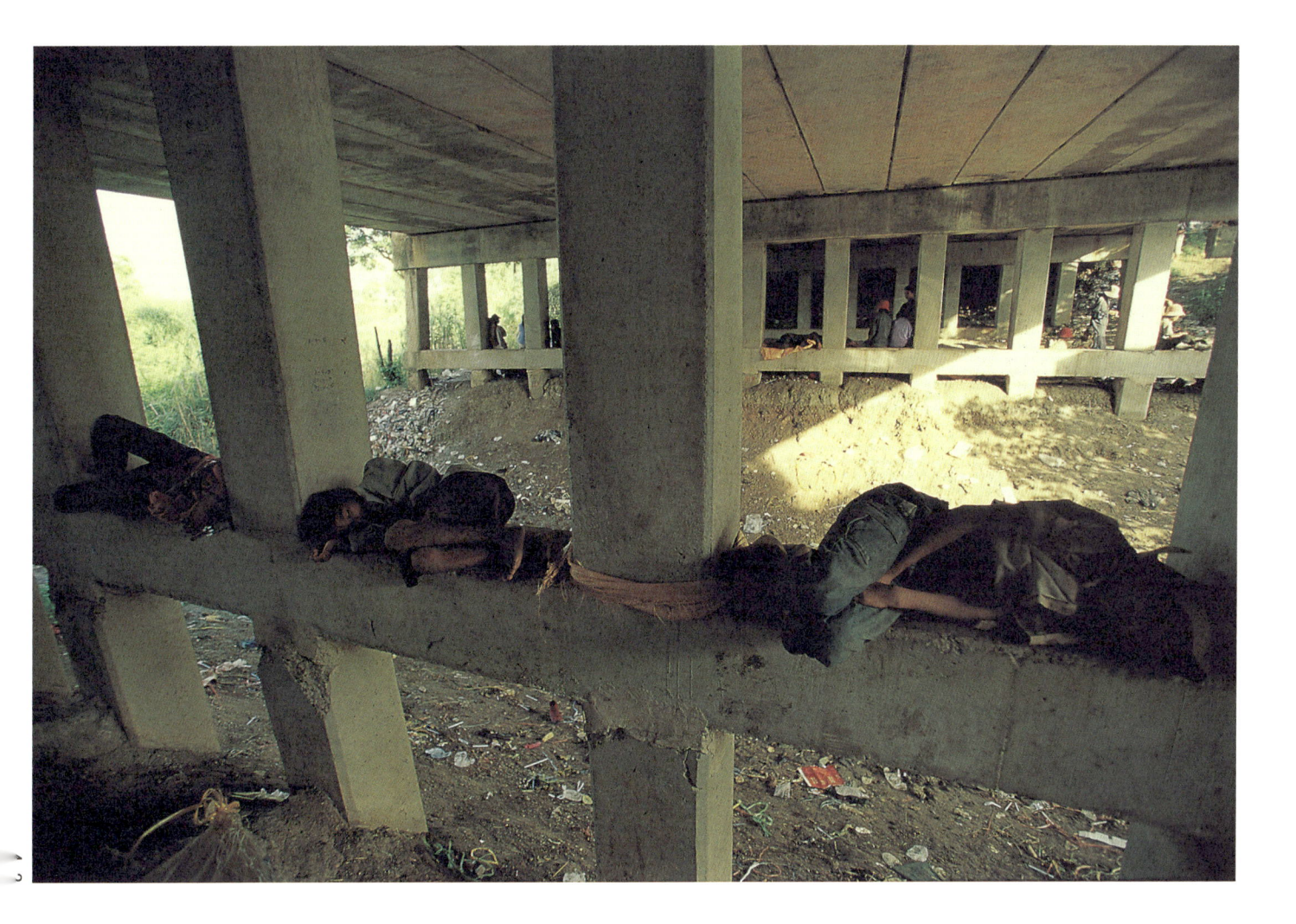

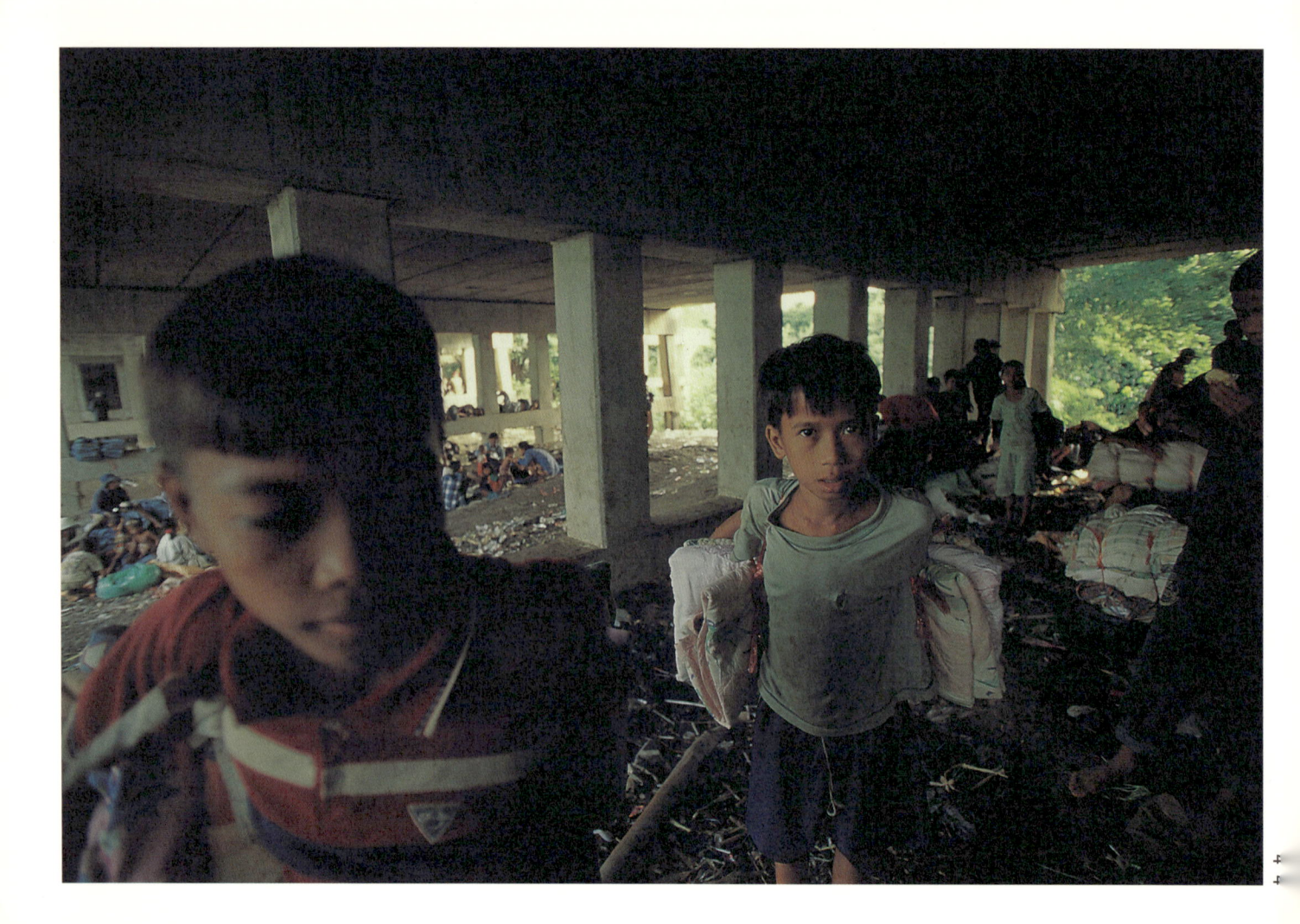

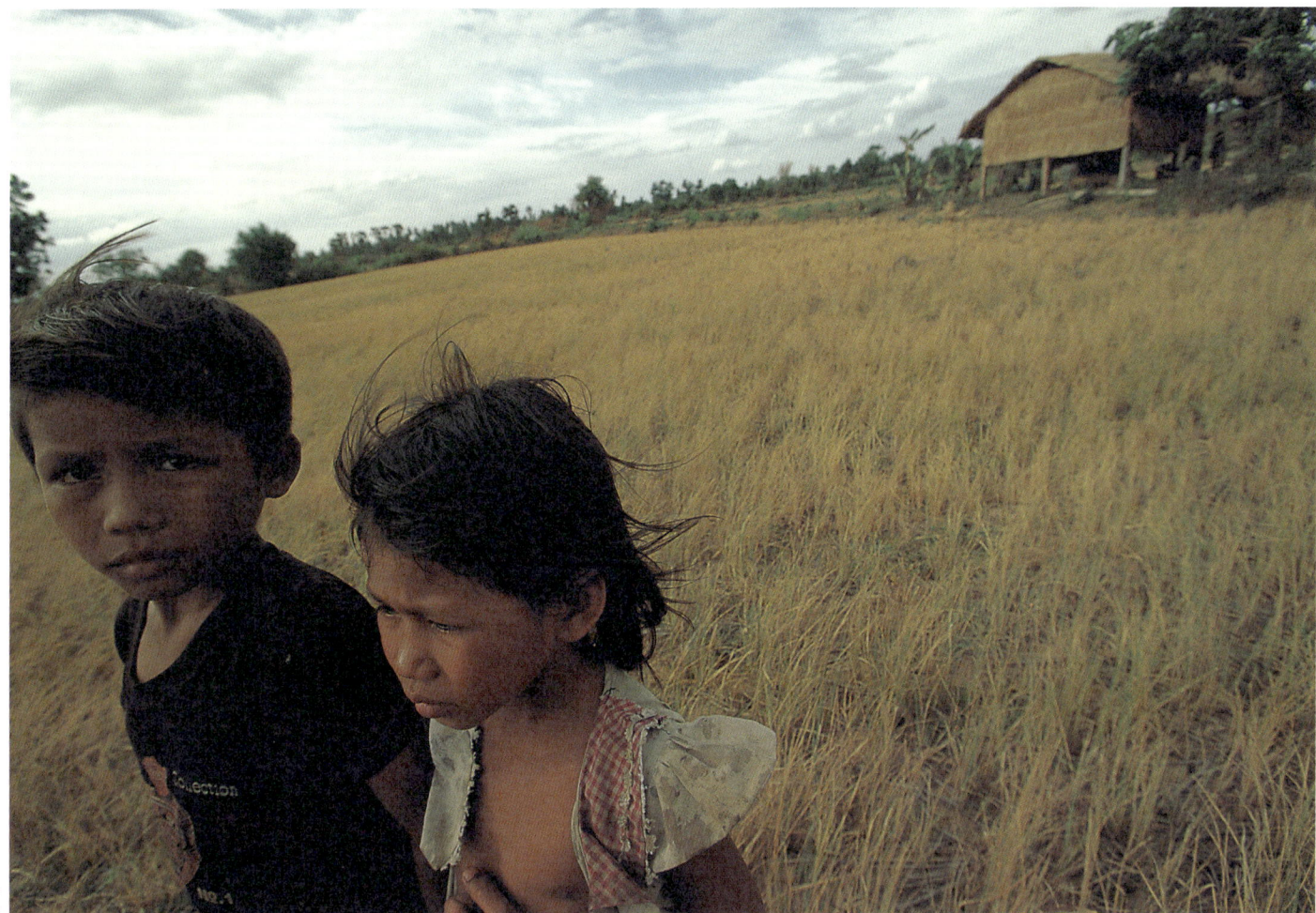

11 リナ

　2003月2月。タイ国境の町パイリンで働くリナは、今年20歳になる。売春宿が密集する一角で、彼女は退屈そうにタバコを吹かしていた。生まれはベトナム国境付近の村だという。

　リナの腕には切り傷がたくさんあった。嫌な客の相手をする時、リナはアンフェタミンと呼ばれるドラッグを吸って気分を高める。そして薬が切れて現実に戻された時、生きているのが嫌になり、腕を切るという。

　「死にたくはないわ。だけど、生きていても地獄だから、死んで楽になりたいと思う」

　女性たちはみな、貧しいがために売られてきた。逃げ出して捕まると、酷い仕打ちを受ける。数軒離れたカラオケバーでは半年ほど前、1人の女性が自ら腕を切り、出血多量で死んだ。体には殴られてできた痣がいくつもあった。警察が来たが、トラブルを恐れた店の主人は、彼らに賄賂を渡した。そして女性の死は、ただの麻薬中毒者の自殺ということで簡単に処理され、調査は何も行なわれず、事件にもならなかった。

11 Lina

In February 2003, I met Lina who was working in Pailin, near the Thai border. She said she would turn 20 later in the year. She absent-mindedly smoked a cigarette on a street corner where several brothels stood close together. She said that she was born in a village near the Vietnamese border.

　There were many cuts in Lina's arm. When she takes an unwanted customer, Lina smokes amphetamines to raise her spirits. When the drug wears off, she returns to reality, a reality she is tired of living. Then she slices her arm.

　"I don't want to die. But even now I am living in hell," she says. She thinks that any death must be easier than her current life.

　The women here were sold to the brothels by their poor families. They could run away but if they are caught, they are treated cruelly. About 6 months ago, one woman sliced her own arm and she bled to death in a karaoke bar a few doors down. There was a cruel bruise on her body where she had been beaten by someone. Though the police came, the owner of bar was afraid of the trouble, so he bribed them. The police ruled the woman's death a mere drug addict's suicide and the investigation ended.

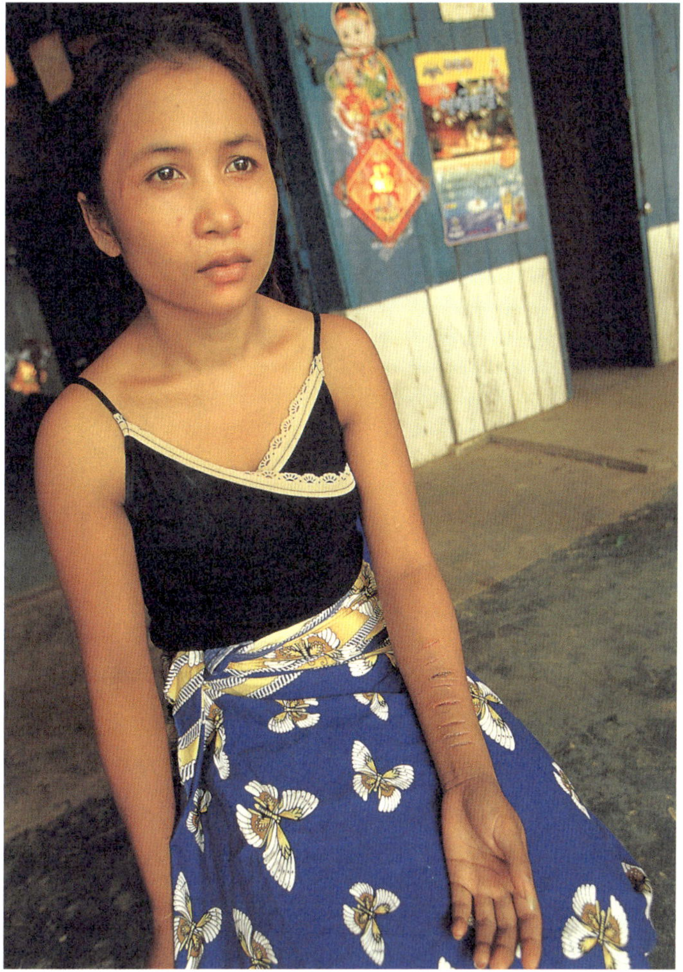

40

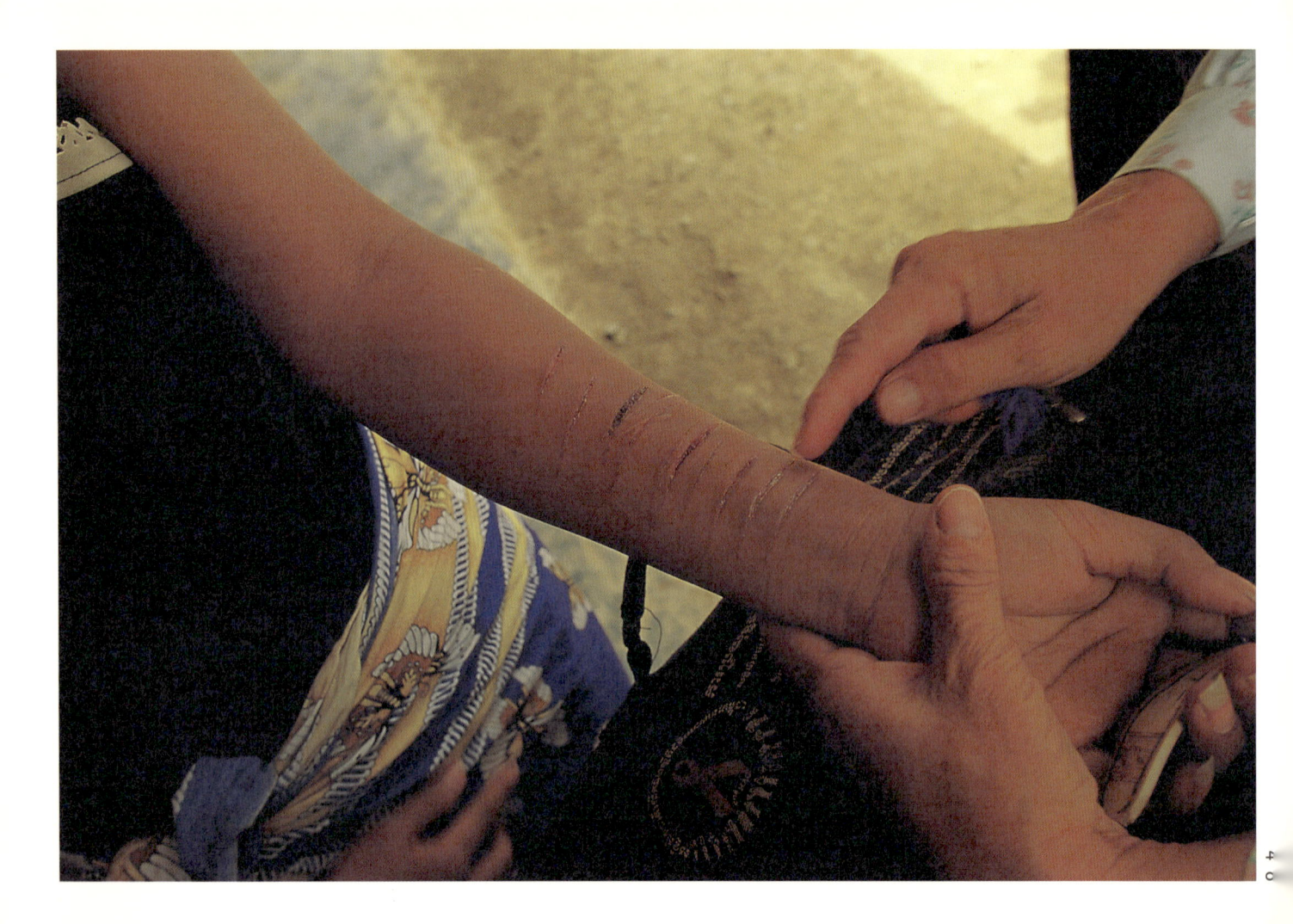

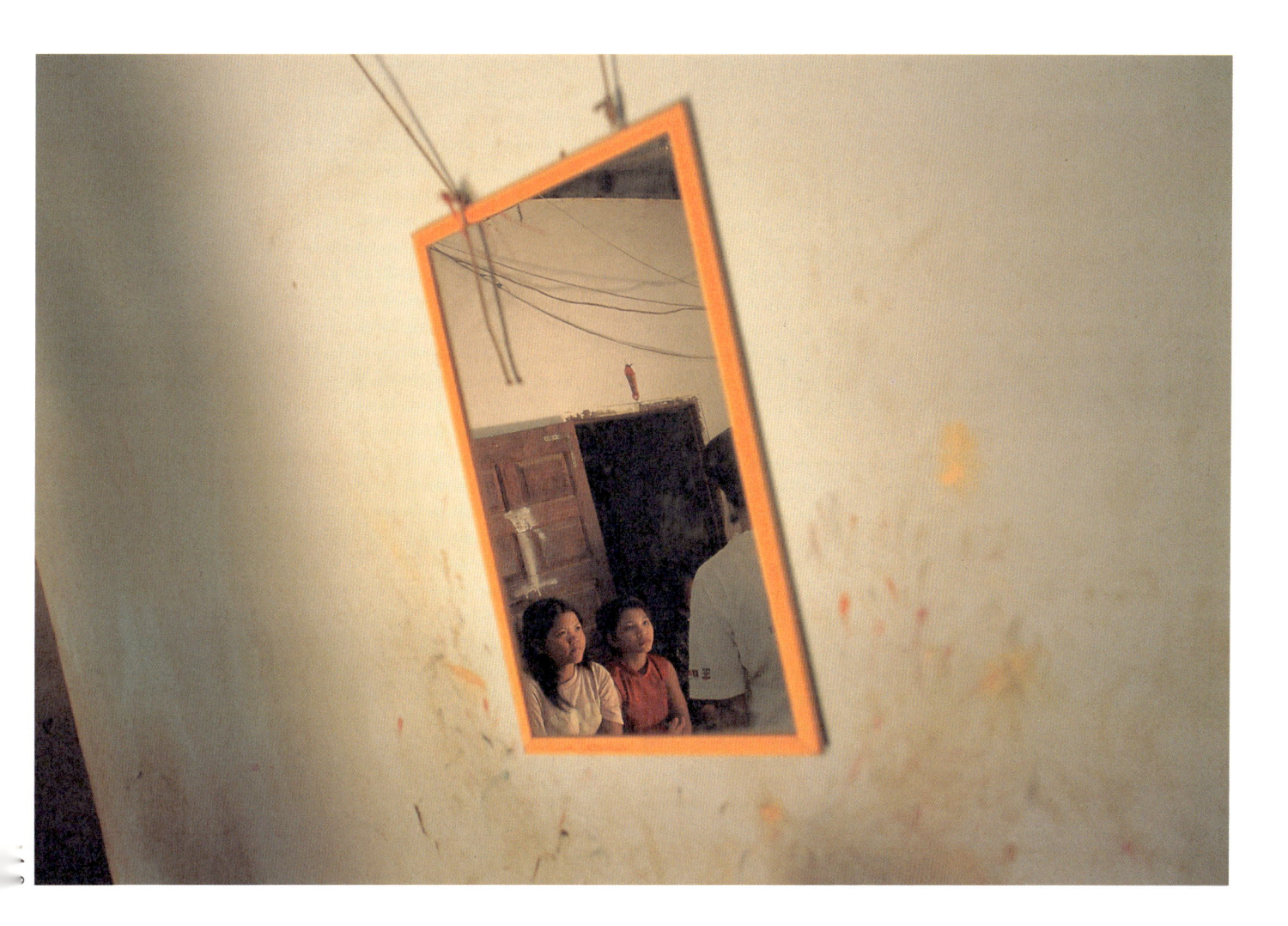

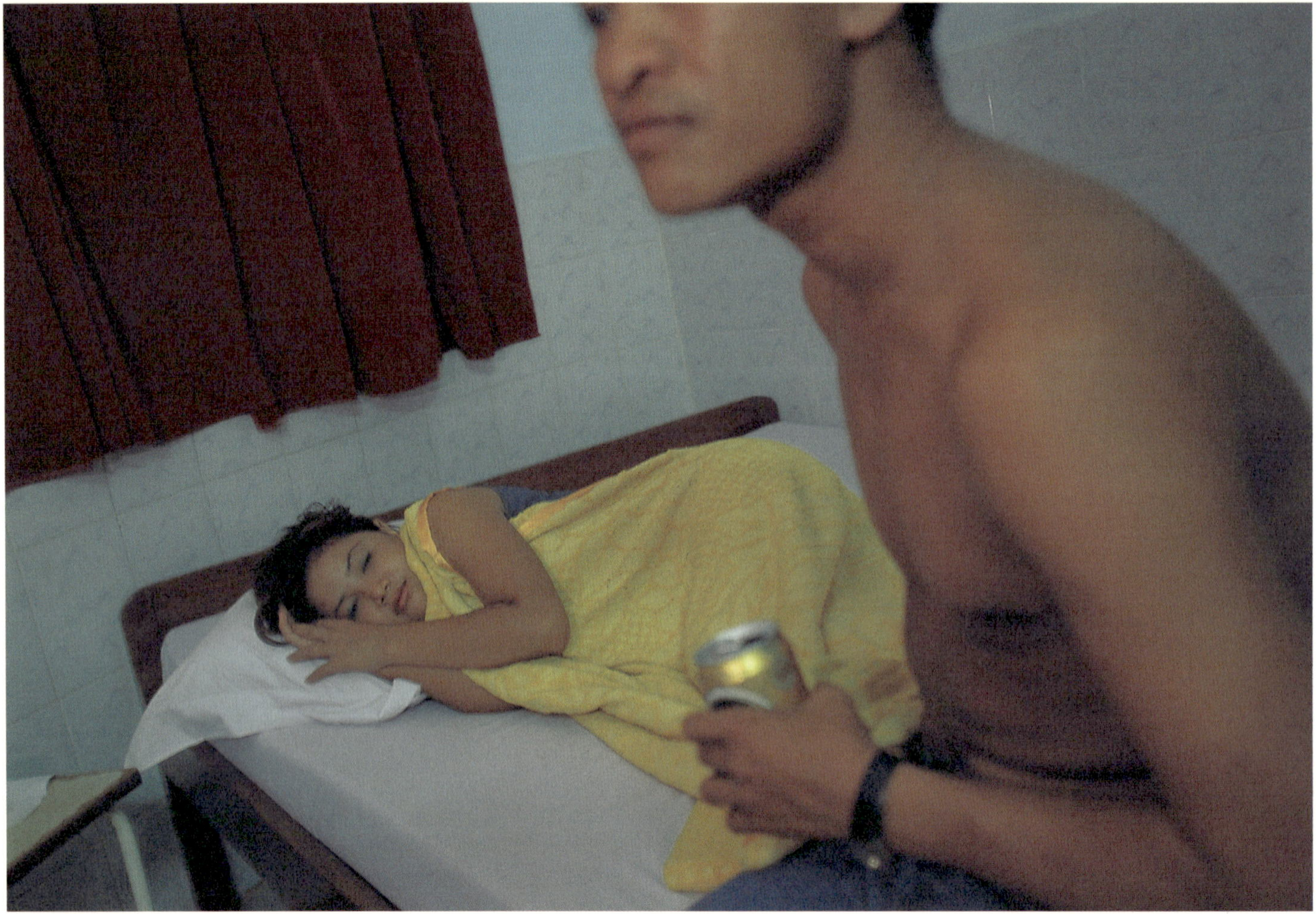

12 ミセス・コンドーム

「まず袋を破りコンドームを取り出す。そしてペニスの根っこをつかむ。そら！やってみなさい！」

2003年2月。バッタンバンの中学校。教室にソフィアング校長の声が響いた。49歳になる彼女は、生徒たちから「ミセス・コンドーム」と呼ばれている。以前は普通の教師だった。しかし、故郷の村で見たエイズの恐怖が彼女を変えた。

「村は貧しく、みな仕事を求めてタイ国境に行きました。しかし90年代後半から、具合が悪くなった人々が、少しずつ村に戻り始めたのです」。それから村で、ばたばたと人が死に始めた。彼女もたくさんの友人をエイズで亡くした。自分に何ができるのかと考え、生徒たちにエイズ教育を始めた。

「政府は何もしてくれない。私たちががんばらないと、この国の未来はないのです」

地元の援助団体「開発と平和を求めるカンボジア女性（CWPD）」の代表リアップさんも、エイズ撲滅を目指す女性の1人だ。パイリンの郊外には、売春宿が集まる小さな村がある。彼女はそこで女性たちにエイズ教育をしている。

リファラル病院の中庭では、この団体のスタッフが毎日、病院にいる女性たちにエイズ教育をしていた。エイズの仕組みを詳しく説明し、女性たちにコンドームを配る。子供たちが、余ったコンドームをふくらませて無邪気に遊んでいた。

12 Mrs. Condom

"Tear the bag open and a take condom out. Then grasp the root of the penis. Try it!"

In February 2003, at a junior high school in Battambang, the voice of principal Sophiang affects a classroom. The 49-year-old woman is called "Mrs. Condom" by her students. She was an ordinary teacher before. But the fear of AIDS she has seen in her village changed her mind.

"My village was poor, so every villager went to the Thai border looking for work. But after the mid-90s, people who got sick returned to the village little by little."

Then, those people started to die in the village. She lost many friends to AIDS. She thought about what she could do, and she started AIDS education for the students.

"The government does nothing," she said. "If we don't do our best, there will be no future in this country."

Ms. Reap is the representative of the local organization Cambodian Women for Peace and Development (CWPD). She aims at AIDS eradication, too. There is a small village where the brothels are concentrated on the suburbs of Poi Pet, near the Thai border. She goes from brothel to brothel, teaching AIDS education to the women there.

Her staff has been teaching AIDS awareness to women every day in the courtyard of Battambang Referral Hospital. The structure of the AIDS disease is explained in detail, and condoms are given to the women. Some bored children who were watching the lecture inflated a left-over condom and played innocently with it.

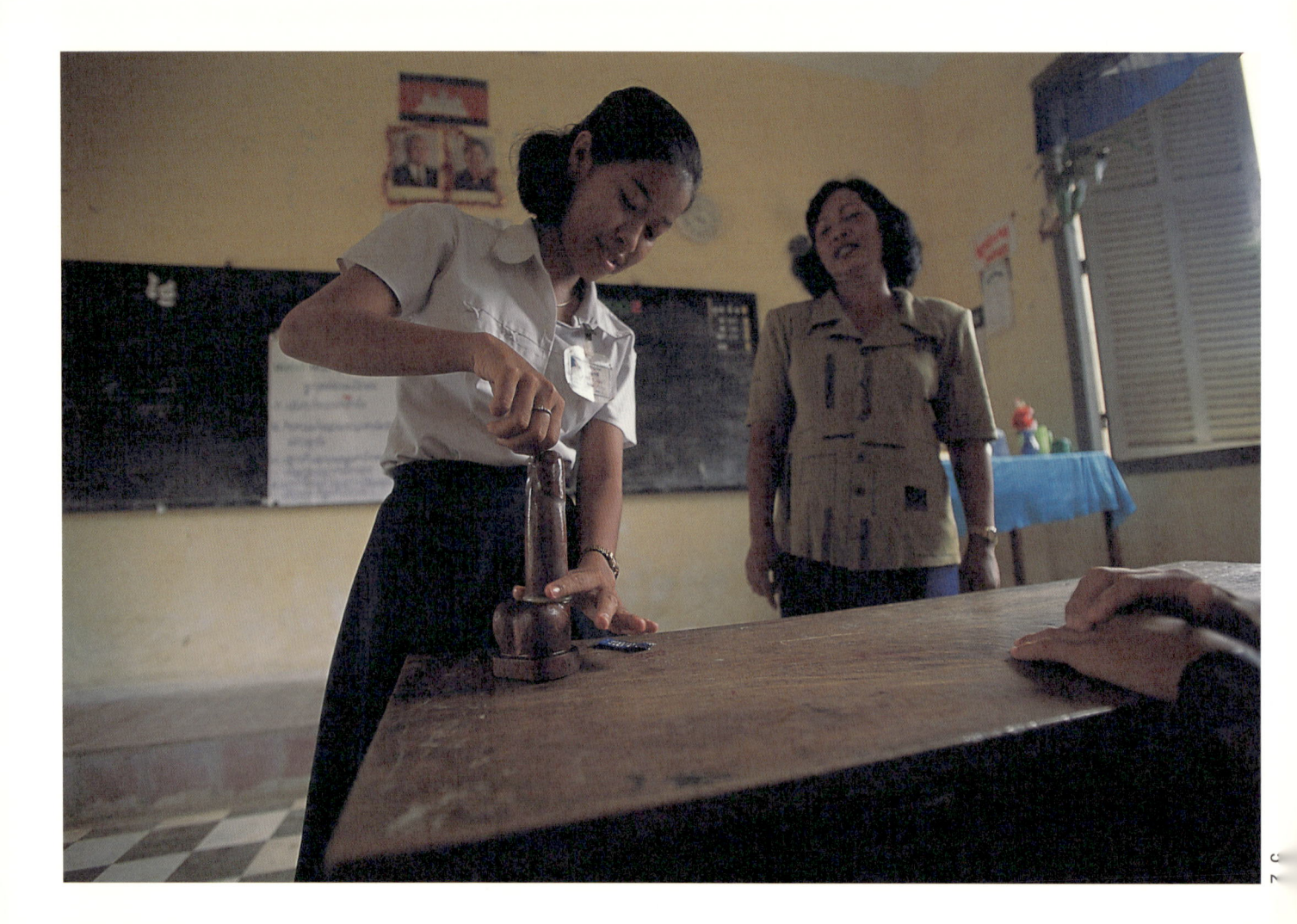

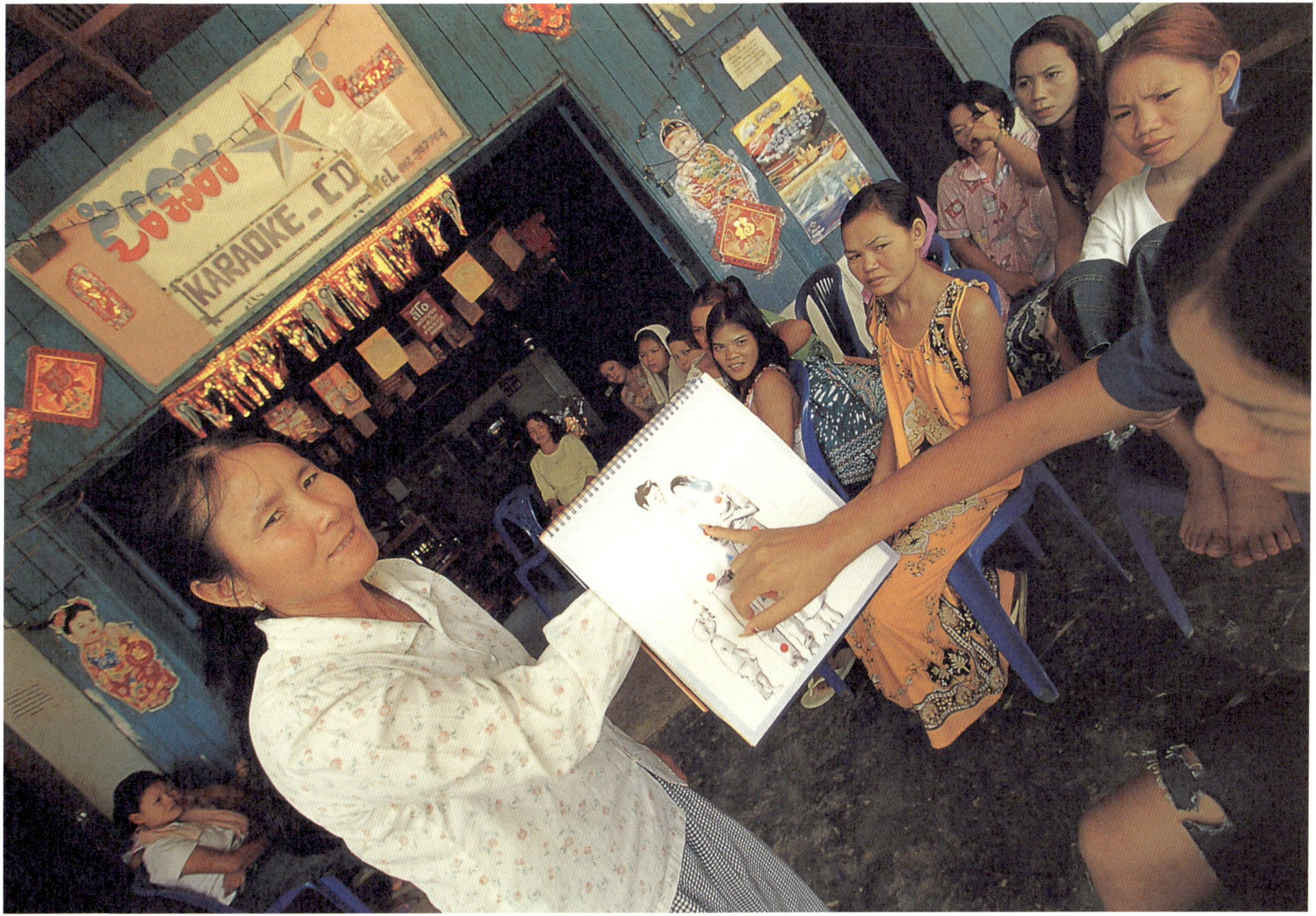
KARAOKE - CD

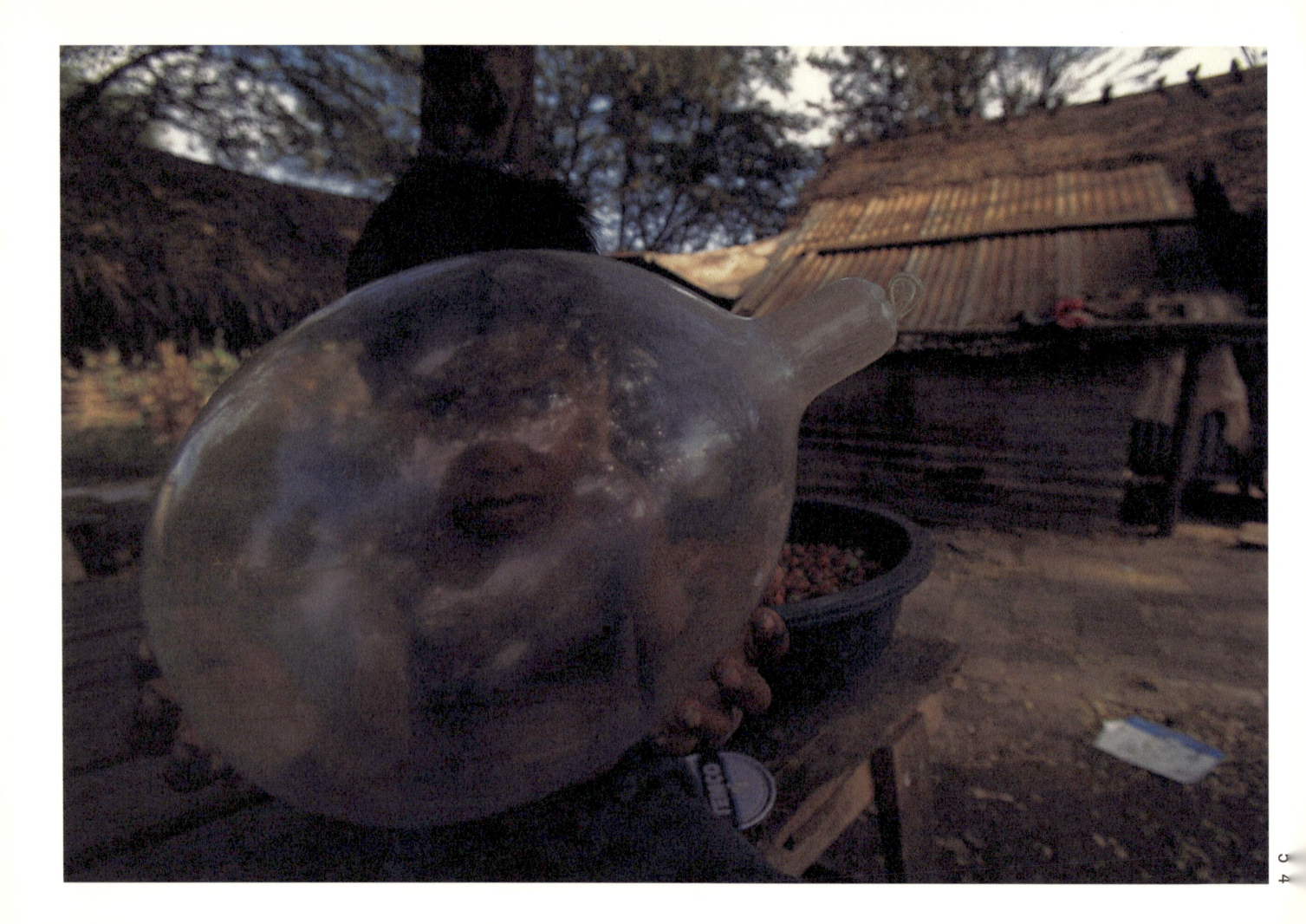

13 カンハ

　2001年4月。スコールが激しく降り、病室の窓から雨が吹き込んでいた。12歳のカンハは、窓際のベッドに横たわっている母に雨がかからないように気をつけながら、お粥を食べさせていた。

　「マエ（お母さん）、もう少し食べる？」

　既に言葉を話す気力もない母親は、黙ってうなずいた。

　母の死はあっけなかった。いつもの通りお粥を少し食べ、薬を飲んだあと、母はベッドで横になった。カンハが洗濯をして戻り、母を見ると、目を閉じたまま眠るように死んでいた。

　カンハの故郷はバンテアイミヤンチェイ州にある。村には帰りたくなかった。母がエイズを発病した時に、村人たちから酷い仕打ちを受けたからだ。

　途方に暮れていた彼女を、病院の駐車場を管理していた親切な家族が引き取ってくれた。午前中は学校に行き、午後は駐車場で働く日々が続いた。

　しかし1年ほど経ったある日、プノンペンの親類がカンハを引き取りに来た。彼女は嫌だと言ったが、親類の女性は半ば強引に連れ去った。その後、カンハから連絡はない。

13　Kanha

　In April 2001, a squall fell so hard that the rain poured in the windows of the epidemic ward.

　Twelve-year-old Kanha protected her mother from the rain as she lay on a bed near a window. While it rained, Kanha fed rice gruel to her mother.

　"Mae (mother), do you want to eat a little more?"

　The mother, who had become too weak to speak, just nodded in silence.

　The mother's death was sudden. She lay down on her bed after eating the rice gruel and taking her medications. Kanha later returned to the room after washing some clothes. She looked at her mother, but she was already dead, her eyes closed just like she was sleeping.

　Kanha's home village is in Banteay Meanchey province. After her mother died, she didn't want to go back to the village. Before, when her mother became sick, the villagers there treated them badly.

　When Kanha's mother died, one kind family who managed a parking lot in the hospital said she could live with them. While there, she went to school in the morning and worked in a parking lot in the afternoon in her new life.

　But after one year, distant relatives from Phnom Penh came to the hospital to take Kanha. Though at first she refused, the relatives eventually coerced her to leave with them. Since then, no one has heard from Kanha.

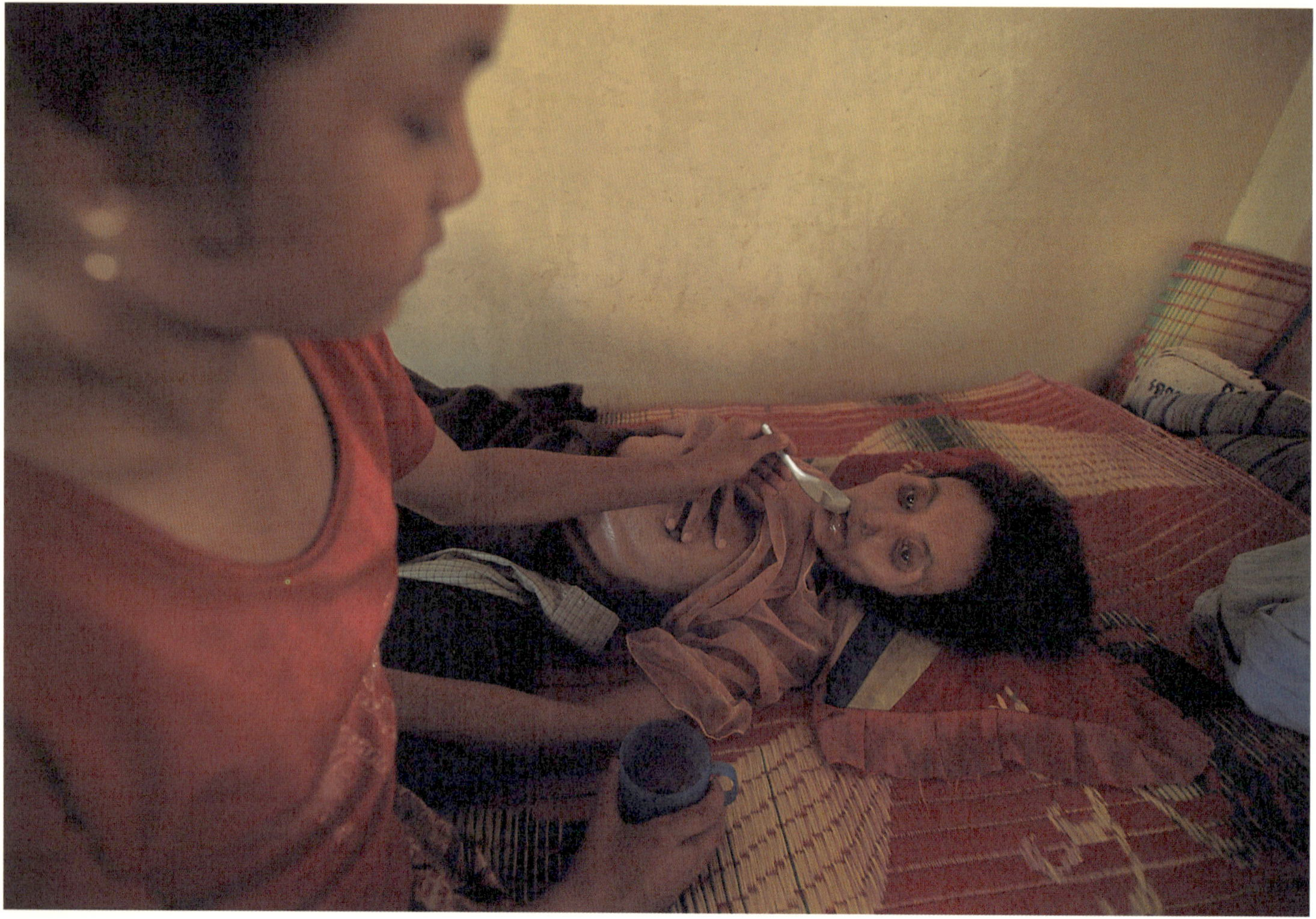

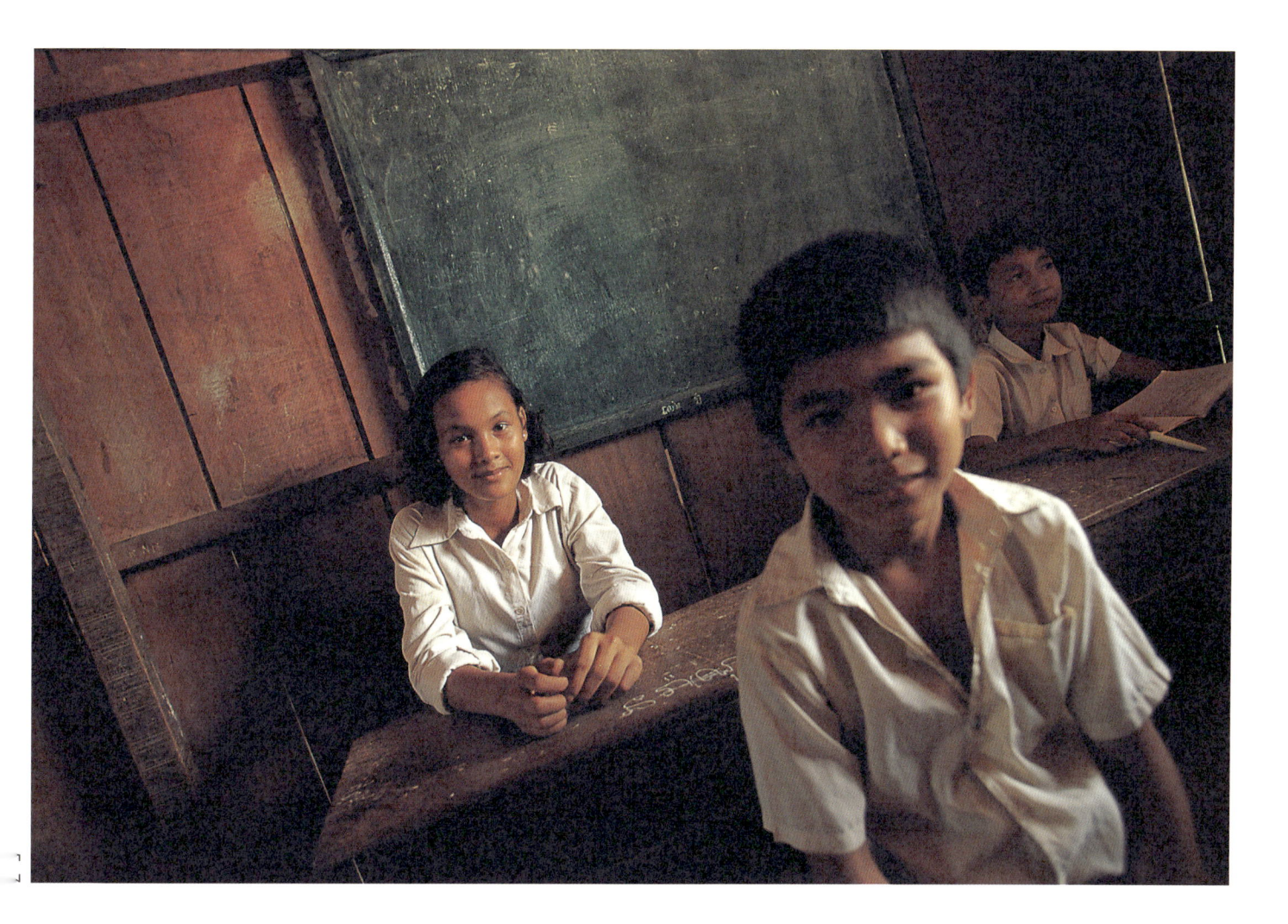

14 チップ

　2002年5月。1人の患者が床に寝かされて、毛布を掛けられていた。

　「おい、あの娘が死んだよ」後ろで誰かが言う。亡くなったのは24歳のチップだった。

　初めてチップを見たのは2ヵ月ほど前だった。エイズを発症した彼女は、1人で病院に来ていた。両親には捨てられた。13歳の時孤児院を抜け出したが、その後売春宿に売られた。彼女はそう言っていた。

　チップの亡骸は近くのお寺に運ばれた。線香を焚いたあと、ガソリンを遺体に振りかけると、瞬く間に遺体は燃え上がった。

　翌日朝早く、僧侶が遺骨を少しばかり集めて寺院に持ち帰った。無縁仏として供養するためだという。

　遺灰は裏庭の野原に捨てられた。放牧された牛がいて、その灰を食べ始めた。誰にもみとられずに死んで、最後は牛の餌になる。僕は写真を撮りながら、これ以上悲しい最期はないと思った。

　雨が降り始め、牛が食べ残した遺灰は雨に打たれ、田園に続く水路に流されていく。チップはゆっくりと土に返っていった。

14 Tip

In May 2002, there was one patient lying on the floor of the epidemic ward covered in a blanket.

"Hey, the girl died already." someone said behind me. The dead patient was Tip, just 24 years old. I first saw Tip about 2 months earlier. She told me her short, tragic story: her parents left her. She escaped an orphanage when she was 13 and, after that, she was sold to a brothel by a trafficker. She got AIDS and came to the hospital alone.

Tip's body was carried to a nearby temple. Incense was lit and her body flared up in an instant from the gasoline sprinkled on her.

Early the next morning, a Buddhist monk collected some of Tip's ashes. He brought them inside the temple for a small memorial service as none of her relatives were there to perform it. The rest of Tip's ashes were thrown away in the backyard of the temple. A cow grazed there, and it began to eat the ashes. Tip was nursed by no one until she died, and in the end she became cow fodder.

While taking pictures, I felt that her death was the saddest ending I had ever seen.

Rain started to fall, and the ashes which the cow left were washed away to a ditch leading to nearby rice fields. And Tip went back to the land slowly.

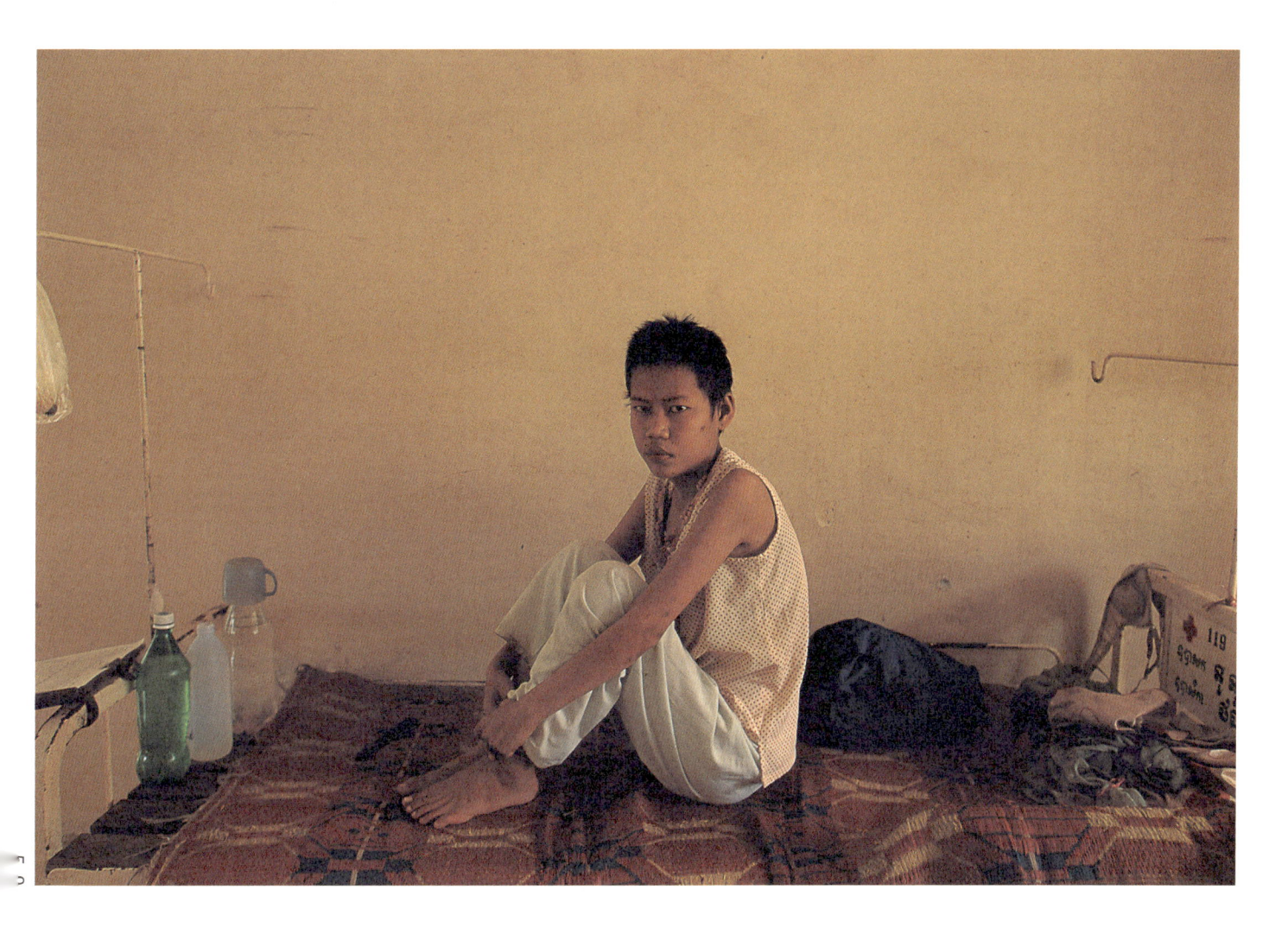

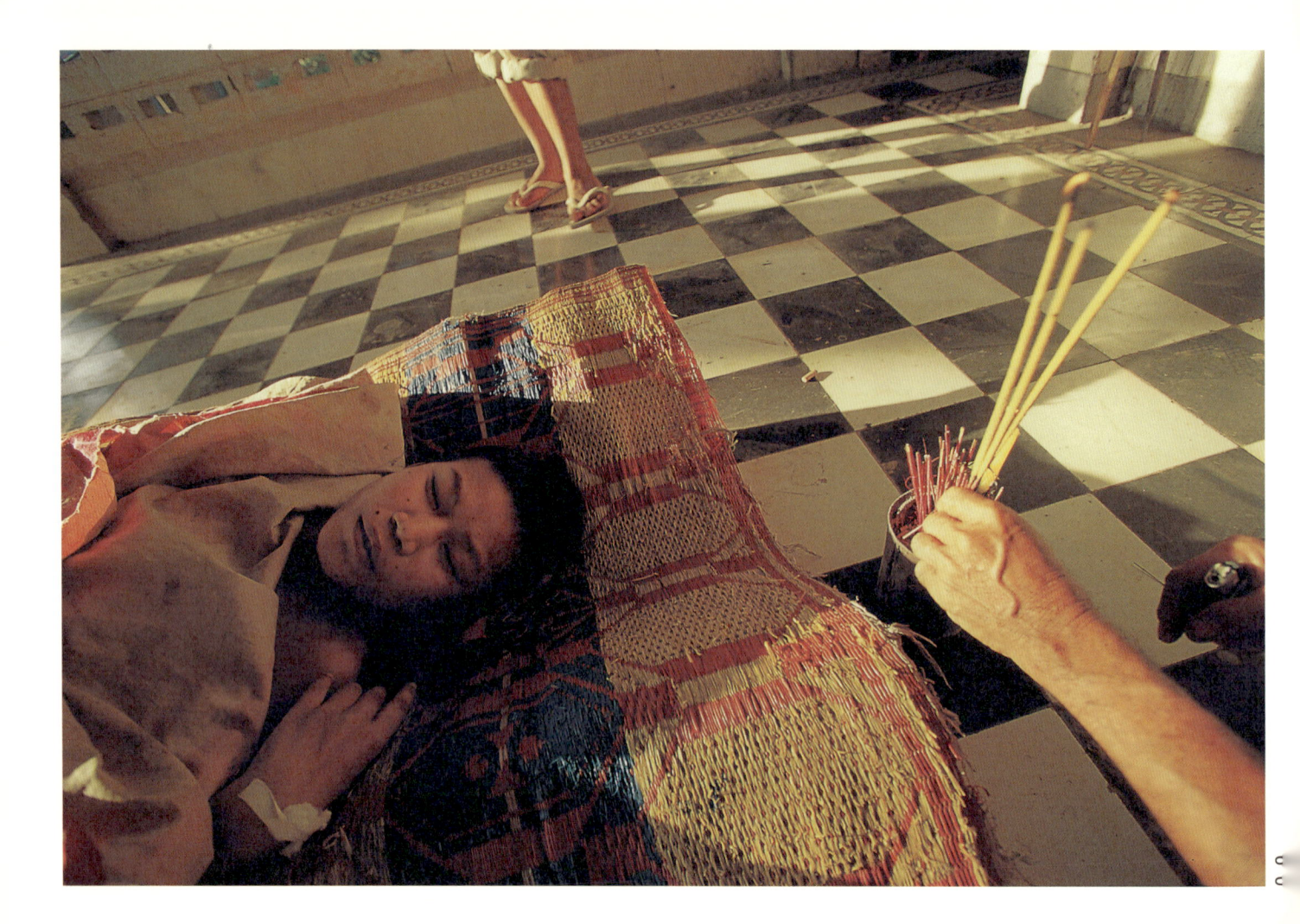

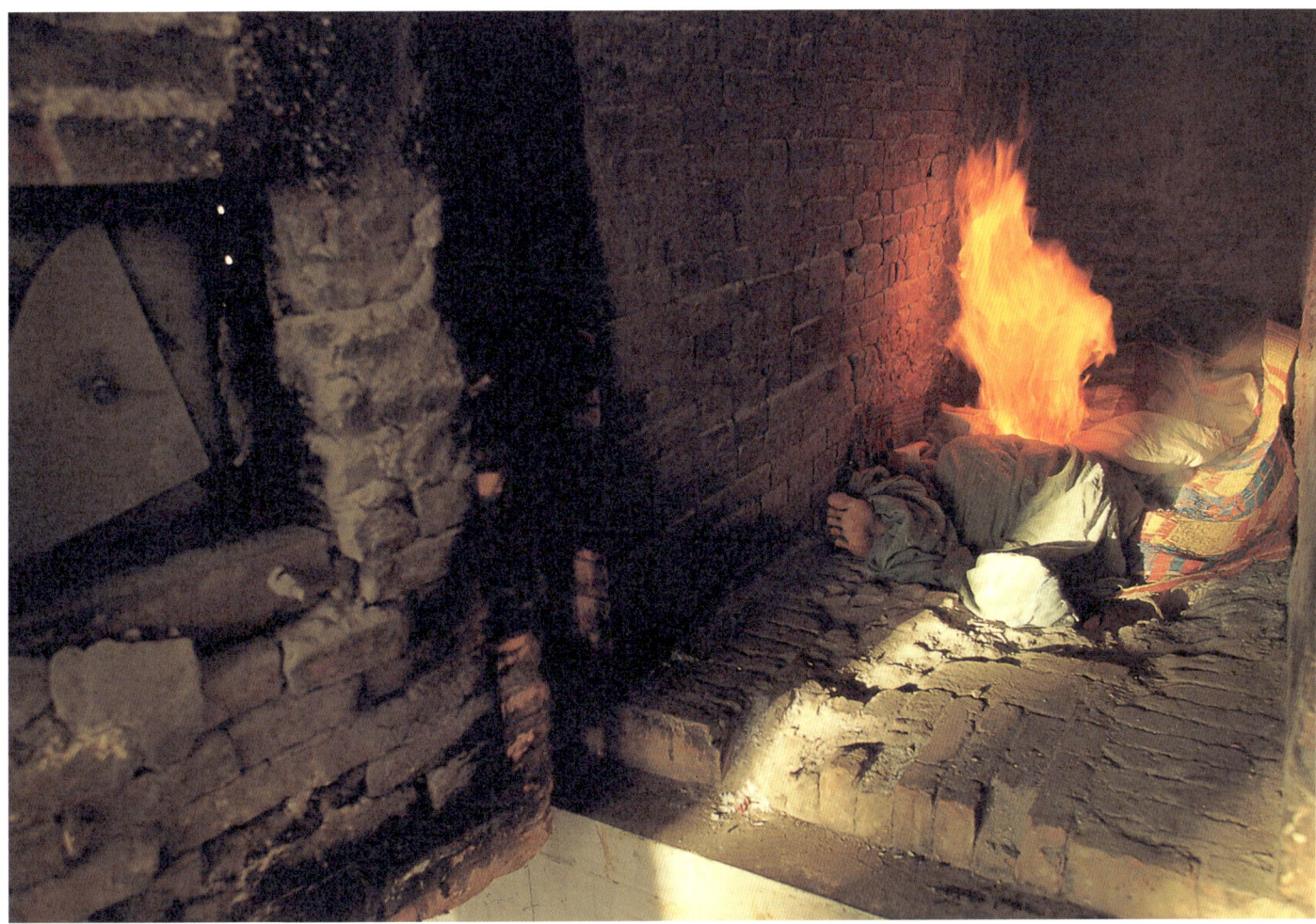

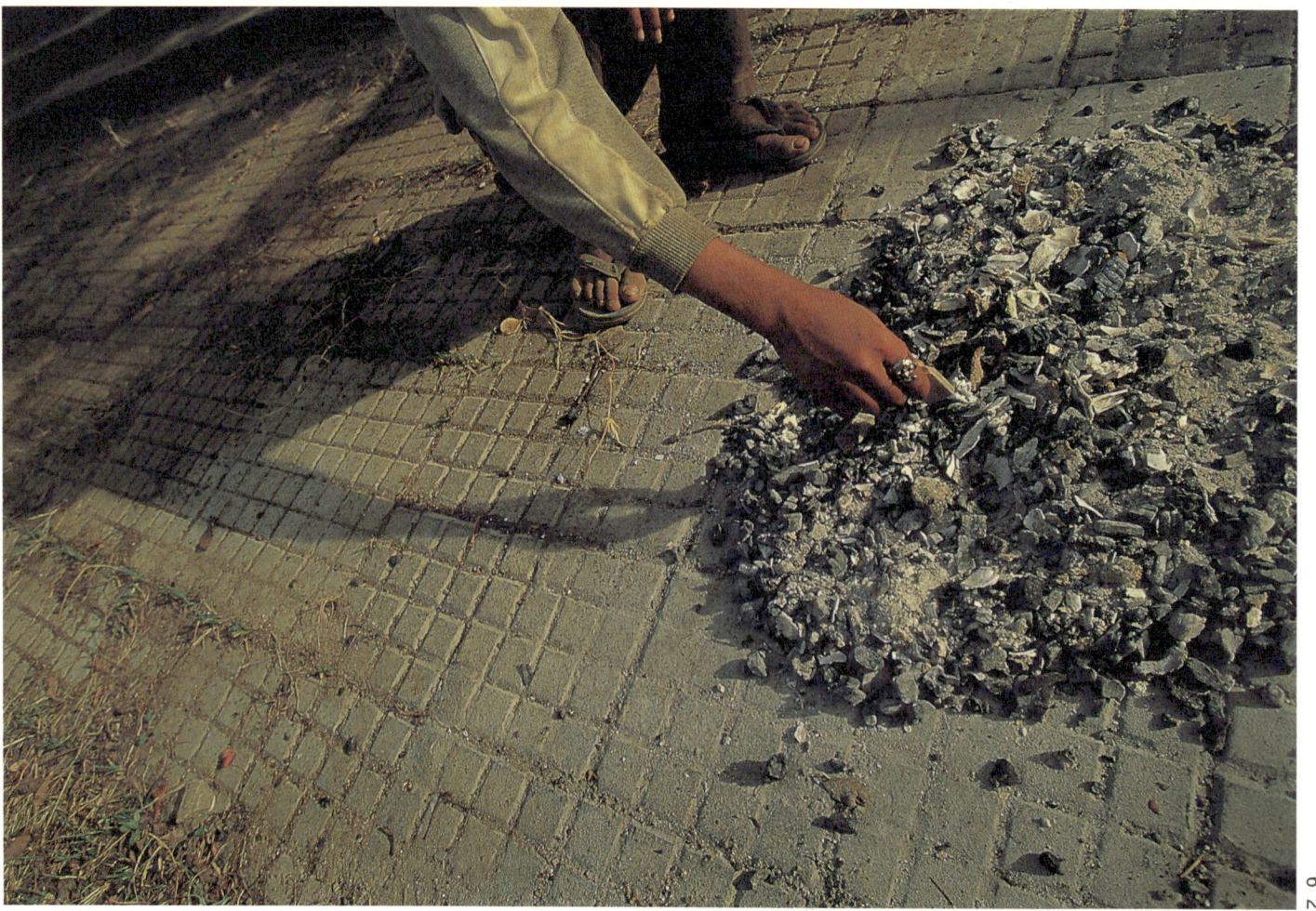

15 ヒム

　2002年6月。まだ日が昇って間もない午前6時過ぎ、ベッドで横になるヒムは、じっと一点を見つめていた。「おはよう」と声をかけると、彼はかすかにうなずいた。

　少しして、僕は土産に持ってきたオレンジを取り出した。そして、ヒムを見ると、目を見開いたまま、瞬きもしない。看護師のニダが彼の腕の脈をとった。しばらくして彼女は首を横に振った。

　ニダの目には涙が浮かんでいた。

　「くやしい。苦しんでいる患者が死んでゆくのを見るのは、本当にくやしい。私たちは患者を助けるために働いているのに、それができないのです」

　職員が来て、かっと見開いていたヒムの目を閉じたあと、遺体を担架に載せて運んでいった。ミノムシのように汚れた毛布で包まれたヒムの遺体は、中庭の物置小屋に置かれた。

　翌日、孤児院に預けられていたヒムの子供が病院にいた。母親は既に夫と子を残して家を出ている。

　茶毘に付す前、亡骸の前で線香を焚いた。薪を割る音が響きわたった。残された子供は、ただひとり立ち尽くしていた。

15 Hym

In July 2002, it was 6 AM and the sun was just rising. Hym was lying on a bed and staring at a speck. He nodded a little when I said to him, "Good morning!" About ten minutes later I gave him some oranges as a gift. He didn't blink, though his eyes were open wide. It was his last moment. A nurse, Nida, tried to measure Hym's pulse. Soon she shook her head. Tears appeared in Nida's eyes.

"It is sad. I really regret when I see a patient, who is suffering, eventually die. We are working to help patients, but we cannot."

A hospital staffer came and closed Hym's eyes, which were still open wide. Then the dead body was put on a stretcher and carried outside. Hym's body was wrapped in a dirty blanket like a cocoon, and was put in a storeroom hut in the hospital courtyard. The next day, Hym's son came to the hospital from a nearby orphanage where he had been left. The child's mother had left home long before.

Before the cremation, an incense stick was kindled in front of Hym's remains. The sounds of men breaking firewood filled the temple grounds. A child who was left alone stood there, quietly.

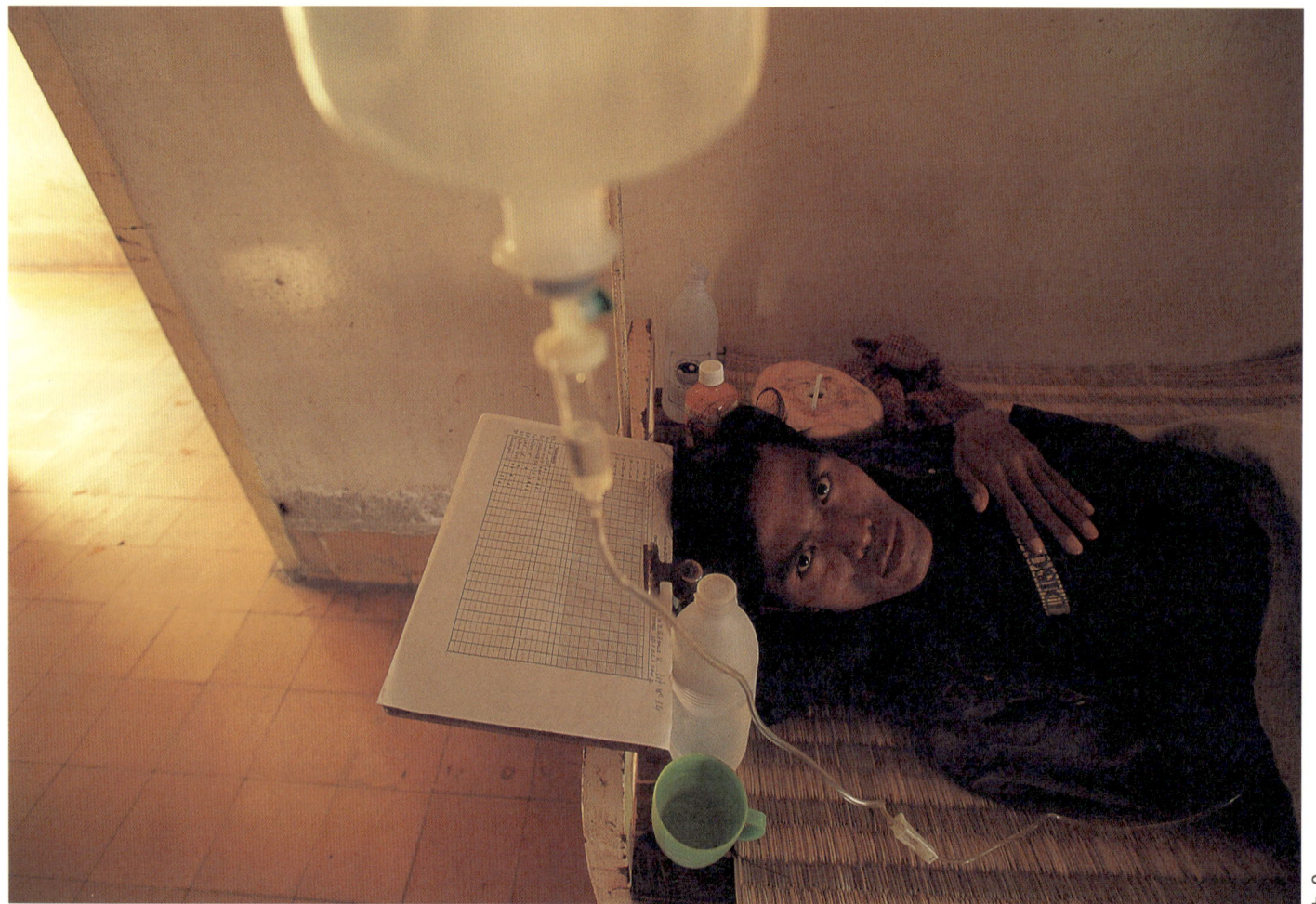

04

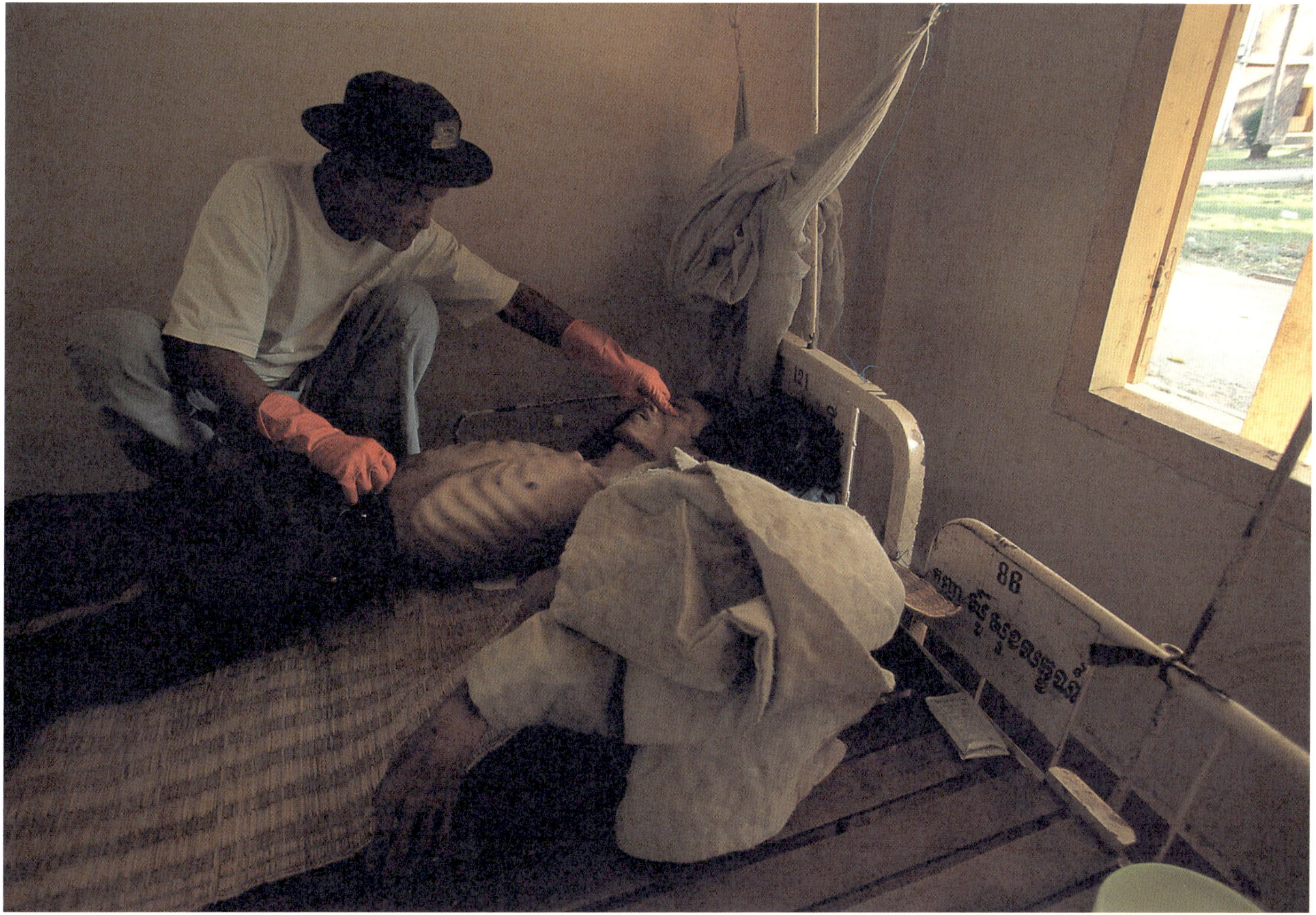

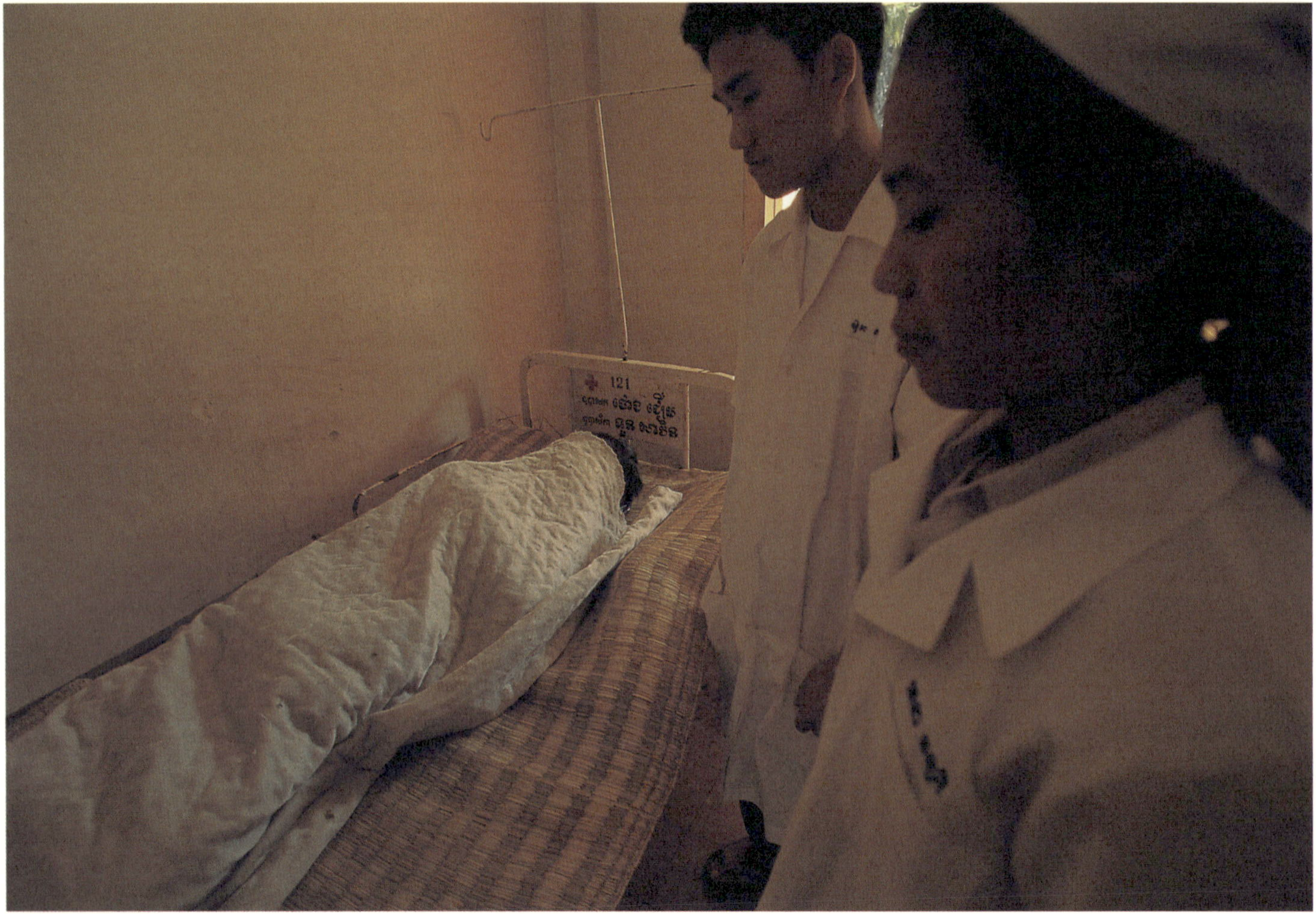
121

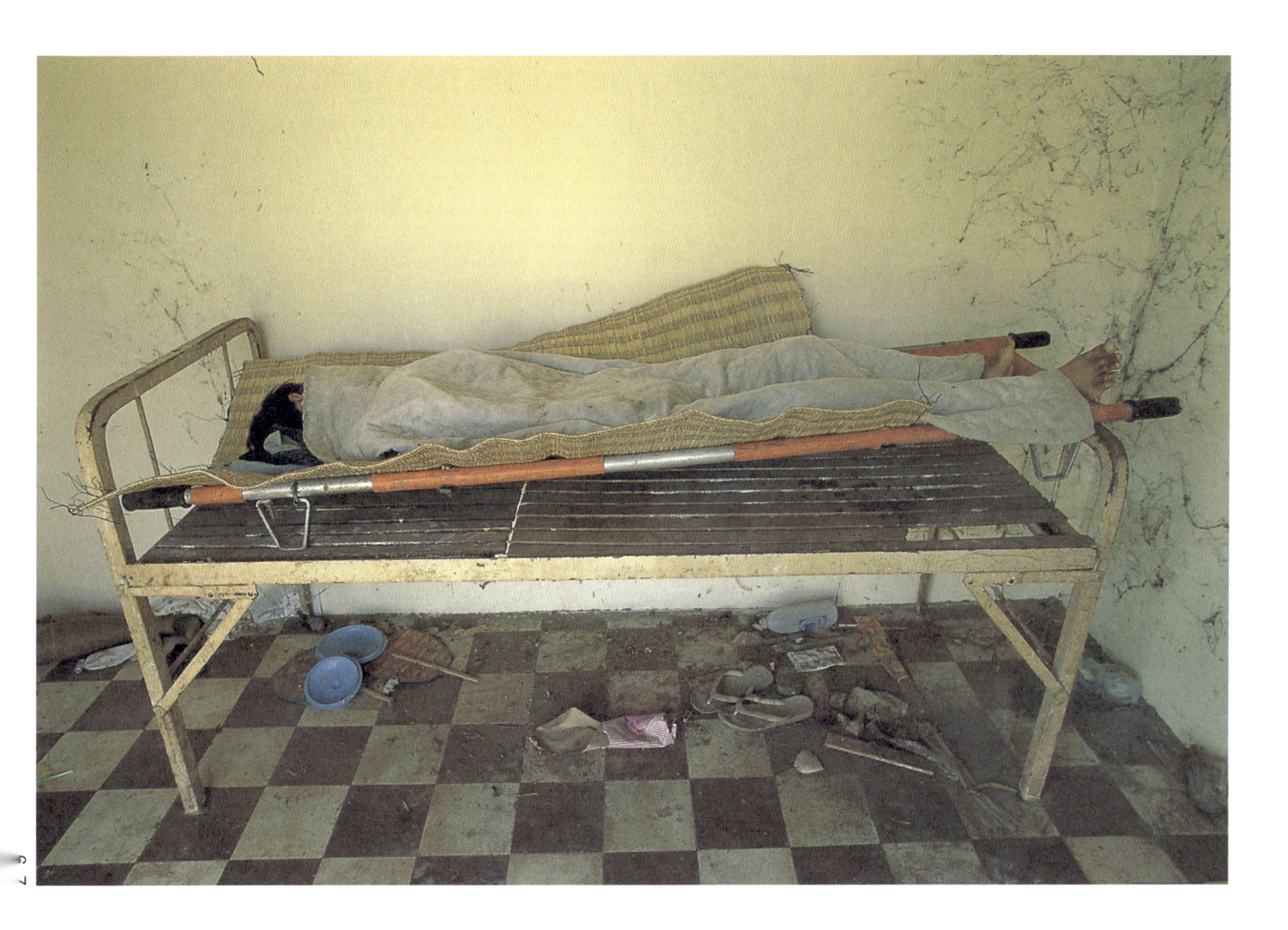

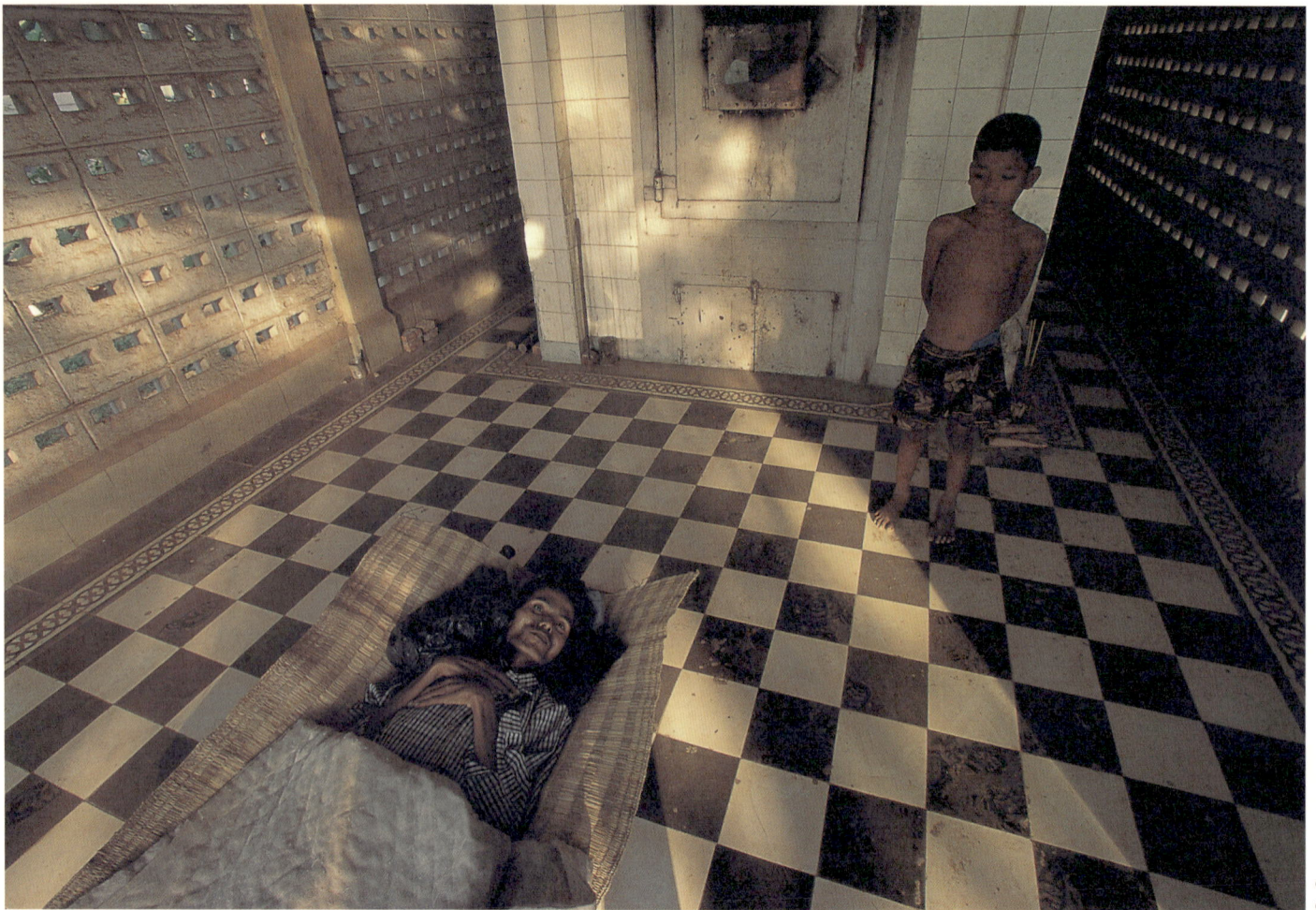

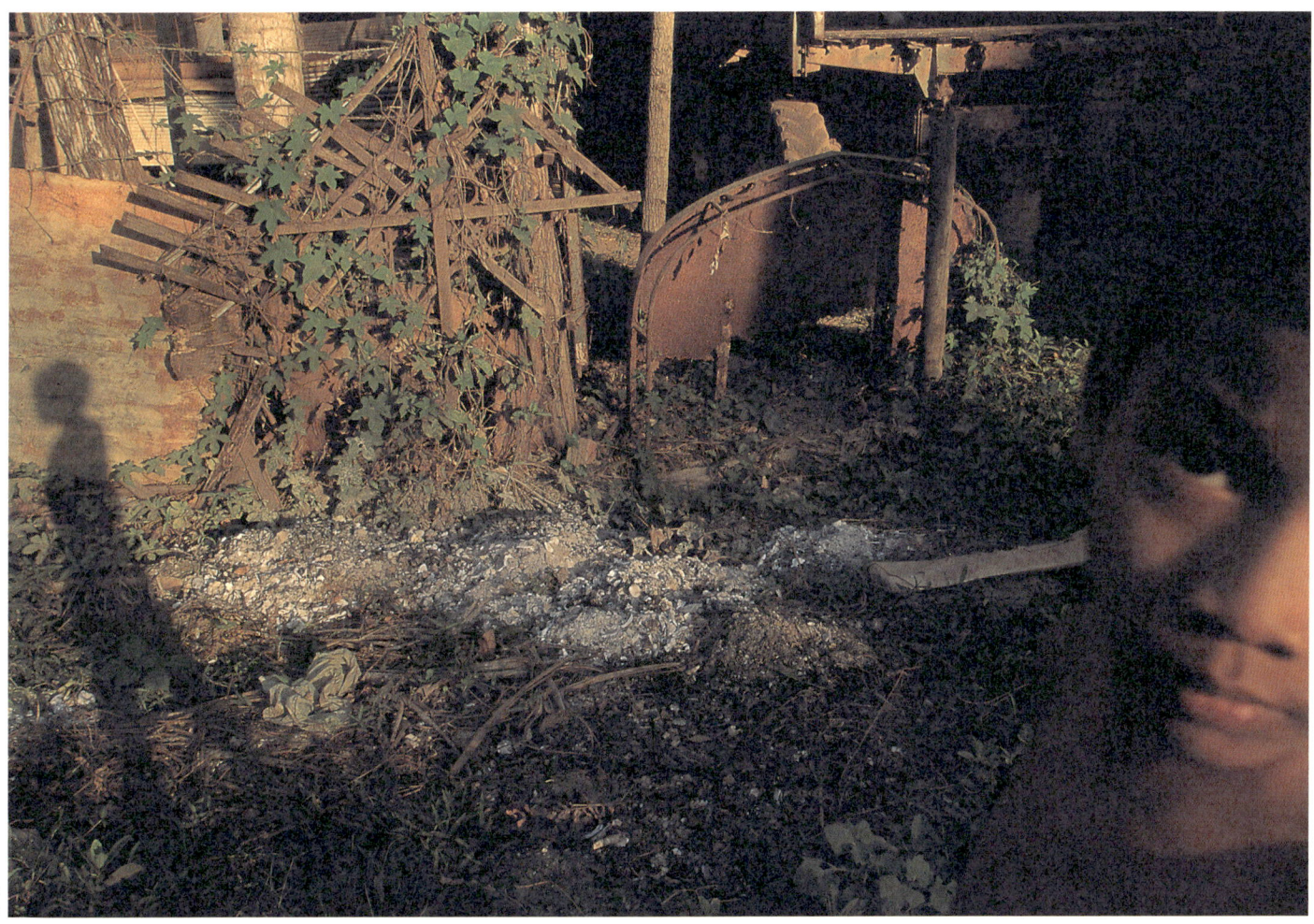

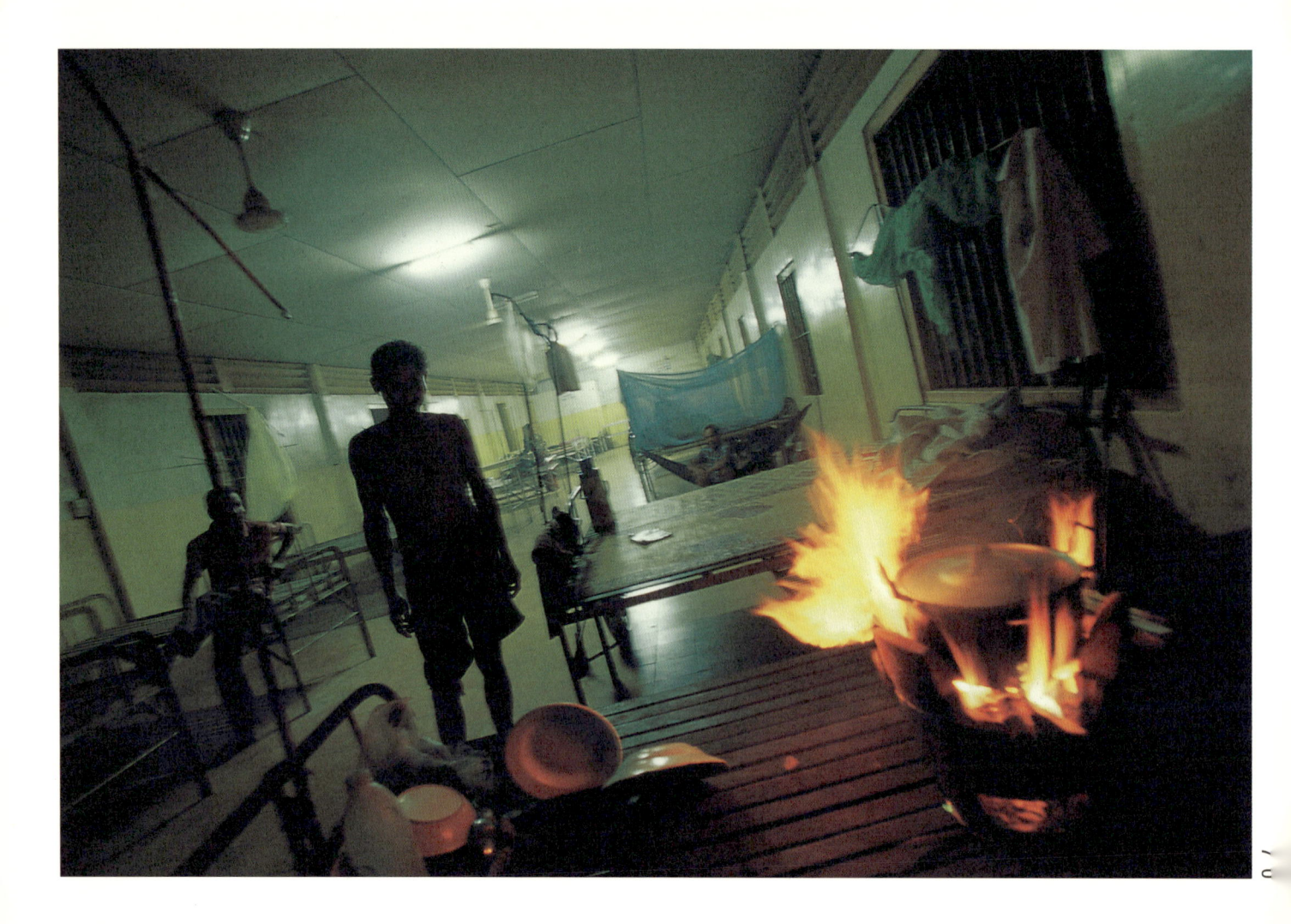

16 スセップ

　感染病棟の所長であるスセップ医師が来て、患者たちの診察を始めた。みな藁をもつかむ思いで、医師の言葉に一心に耳を傾けている。「娘を助けて」と泣いている母親がいた。生きながら地獄のような苦しみに耐えている患者たちは、みな貧しく、絶望の淵で生きている。それは内戦当時に見た光景と同じだった。
　「今、エイズという第２の内戦が、カンボジアを襲っているのです。患者たちを助けたい。何かあなたにできることはありませんか」
　診察を終えたスセップ医師が言う。僕は答えた。
　「写真を撮って、この現状を人々に伝えること。それが僕のできることです」
　医師はしばらく患者たちを見つめ、そして言った。
　「わかりました。私は患者たちに希望を持たせたい。あなたは写真を撮って、人々に伝えてください」
　写真で何ができるのか、わからない。しかし、伝えることで、患者や家族たちの苦しい現状は変わるかもしれない。僕は写真の力を信じたかった。2001年３月18日。この日から、エイズと闘う人々をカメラで追う日々が始まった。

16 Sutthep

Every morning, Doctor Sutthep, chief of the Battambang hospital epidemic ward, conducts medical examinations of everyone in his care. All patients hear the single-minded desire in the doctor's words to grasp at any straws to save their lives. At one bed, a mother weeps and repeats, "Help my daughter." All patients live with the hellish pains of being poor, and they all live in the depths of despair. The scene was the same as what I regularly saw during the civil war.

"The second civil war is AIDS, attacking Cambodia now," says Dr. Sutthep. "I want to help patients. Is there anything you can do for them?" he asks me after finishing his daily examinations.

And I answered.

"I can take photographs and tell people about the actual situation. That is all I can do."

The doctor stared at the patients for a while, and then he said, "I understand. I want patients to have hope. You take a picture, and please tell the people."

But what photograph can make a difference? I had no concrete answer. The actual situation is hard for the patients and their families. But it may change by telling their stories to people out in the world. I want to believe in the power of photography. I met Dr. Sutthep on March 18th, 2001, and from that day I have photographed people who are fighting AIDS.

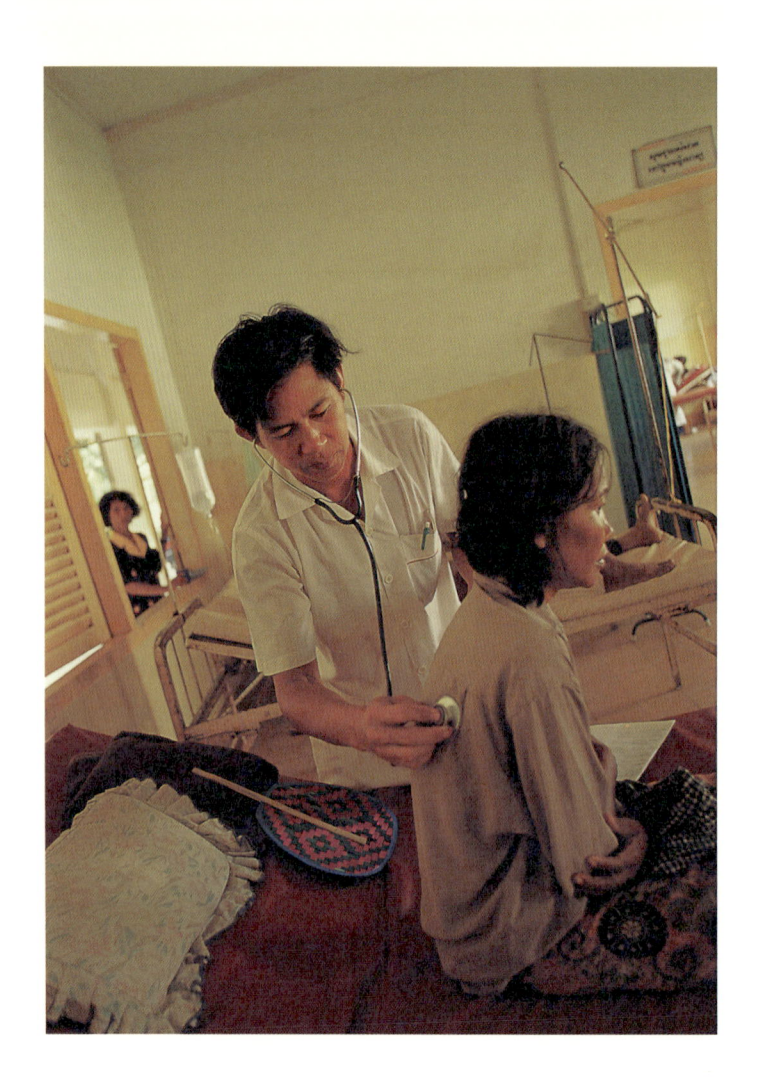

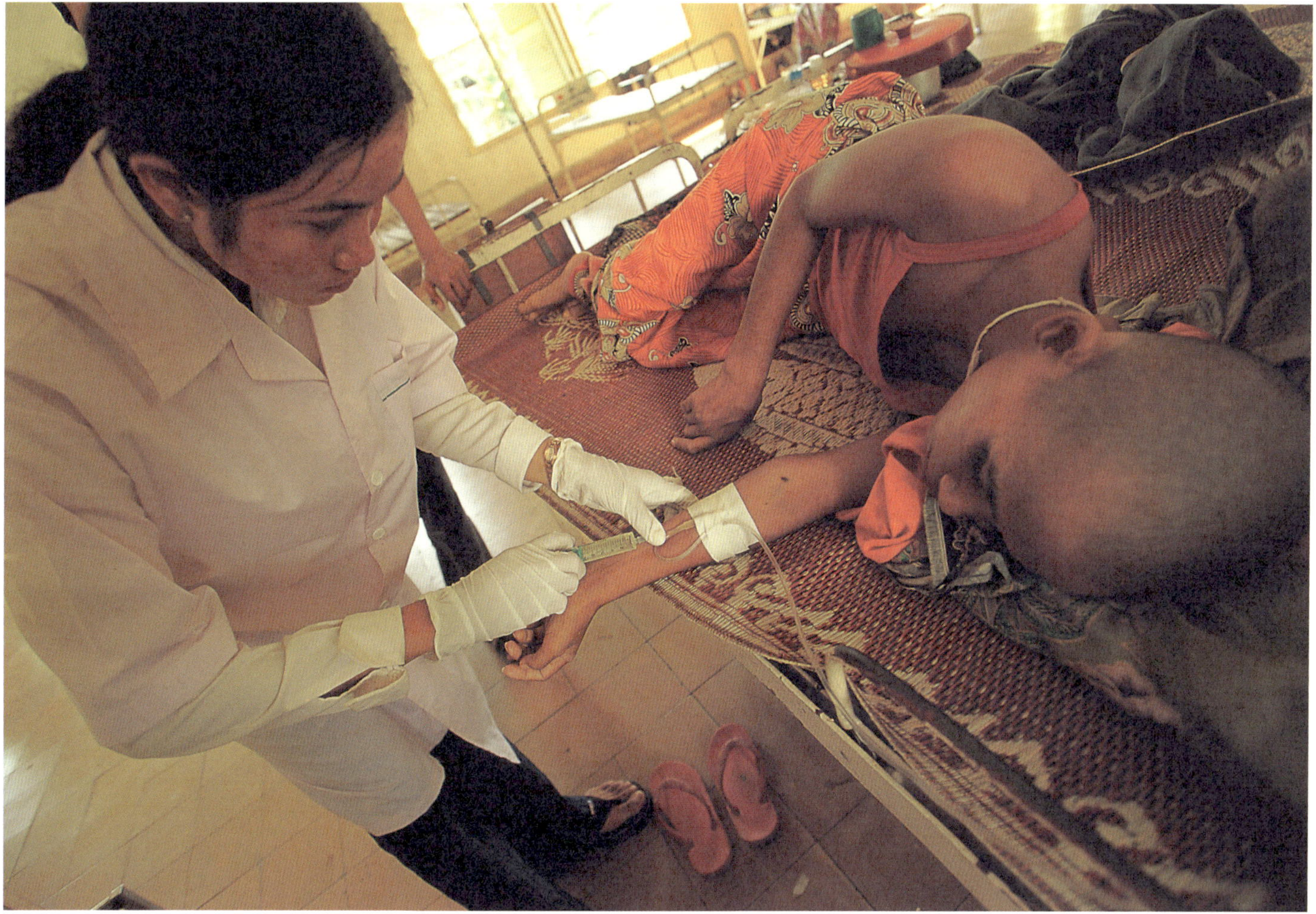

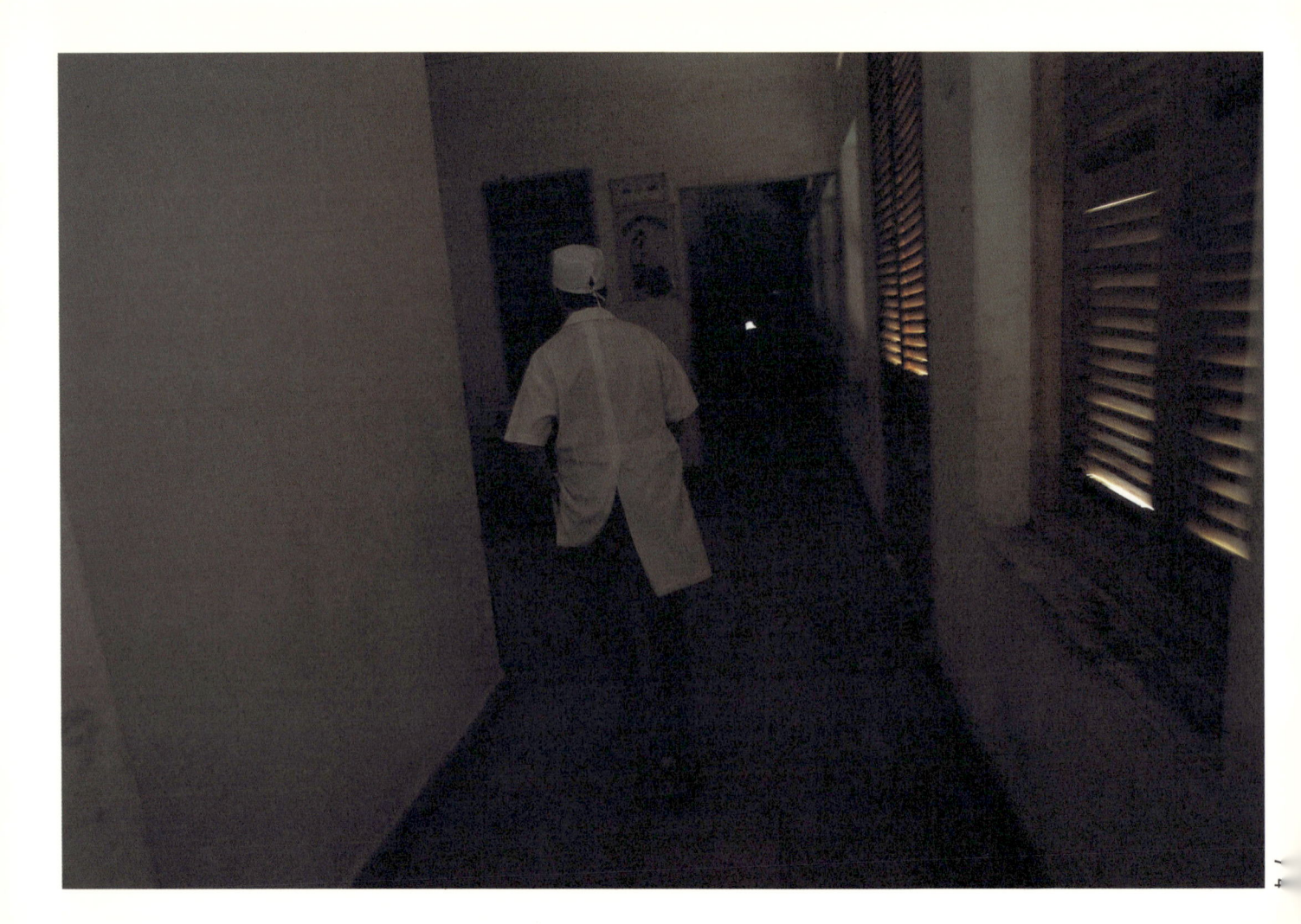

17 セリ

　セリと初めて会ったのは2002年8月だった。エイズ末期の彼女の髪は抜け落ち、母親のヨーンが寄り添うように彼女を看病していた。「娘が元気だった頃の写真です。セリはとてもきれいな子でした」ヨーンは大切そうに、1枚の写真を袋から取り出して僕に見せた。セリには3人の子供がいた。十数年間政府軍兵士として戦った夫は、既に3年前エイズで死んだという。そして半年後の2003年2月、セリは自宅で息を引き取った。残された3人の子供たちは孤児院に送られた。

　2003年3月。バッタンバン市内から1時間ほど離れた畑の中にある小さな孤児院に子供たちを訪ねると、長女のラッキャナーと次男のヴィツ、そして長男のビィティがいて、懐かしそうに僕を見た。その1年後、長男のビィティは孤児院を出て、僧侶となった。寺院にはエイズ患者の施設があり、16歳の彼は患者たちを支えながら、僧侶としての修行を積んでいる。10歳の長女ラッキャナーは現在、シエムリアップにある孤児院で暮らしている。「将来は学校の先生になりたい」施設を訪れると、はにかみながら彼女はそう言った。バッタンバンに残された次男のヴィツは今年13歳になる。両親をエイズで亡くした彼は、「医師になりたい」と語った。エイズ孤児たちの悲しみは計り知れない。孤独に耐えながら、しかしみな夢と希望を持って、今も精いっぱい生きている。

17 Seri

I first met Seri in August 2002, in the epidemic ward of the Battambang hospital. She was in the terminal stages of AIDS and her hair had fallen out. Seri's mother Yoan lay next to her on the small bed as she cared for her daughter.

　Yoan showed me a photo and said, "This picture was taken when my daughter was young. Seri was a beautiful girl."

　Seri had three children, Vuthy, Vithu, and Racanna. Her husband had been a government army soldier for 10 years, but he died from AIDS about 3 years ago. Six months after I met her, Seri finally died from AIDS at her home. Her three children were left alone, and they were sent to an orphanage.

　In March 2003, I visited their small orphanage surrounded by rice fields, about 4 hours from Battambang city. There I met the daughter, Racanna, second son, Vithu, and elder son, Vuthy. They looked to me as an old, familiar face.

　One year later, the elder son, Vuthy, left the orphanage and became a Buddhist monk at age 16. There is a facility for AIDS patients in his temple, and he helps them with traditional Buddhist teachings.

　Racanna, 10, stays in an orphanage in Siem Reap province now. When I visited her, she said shyly, "I want to be a school teacher in the future."

　Vithu was left alone in the orphanage in Battanbang. He became 13 in 2004. He who lost his parents to AIDS told me, "I want to be a doctor."

　The sorrow of the AIDS orphans is immeasurable. Their lives bring great loneliness, but they fight that loneliness with big dreams and hopes.

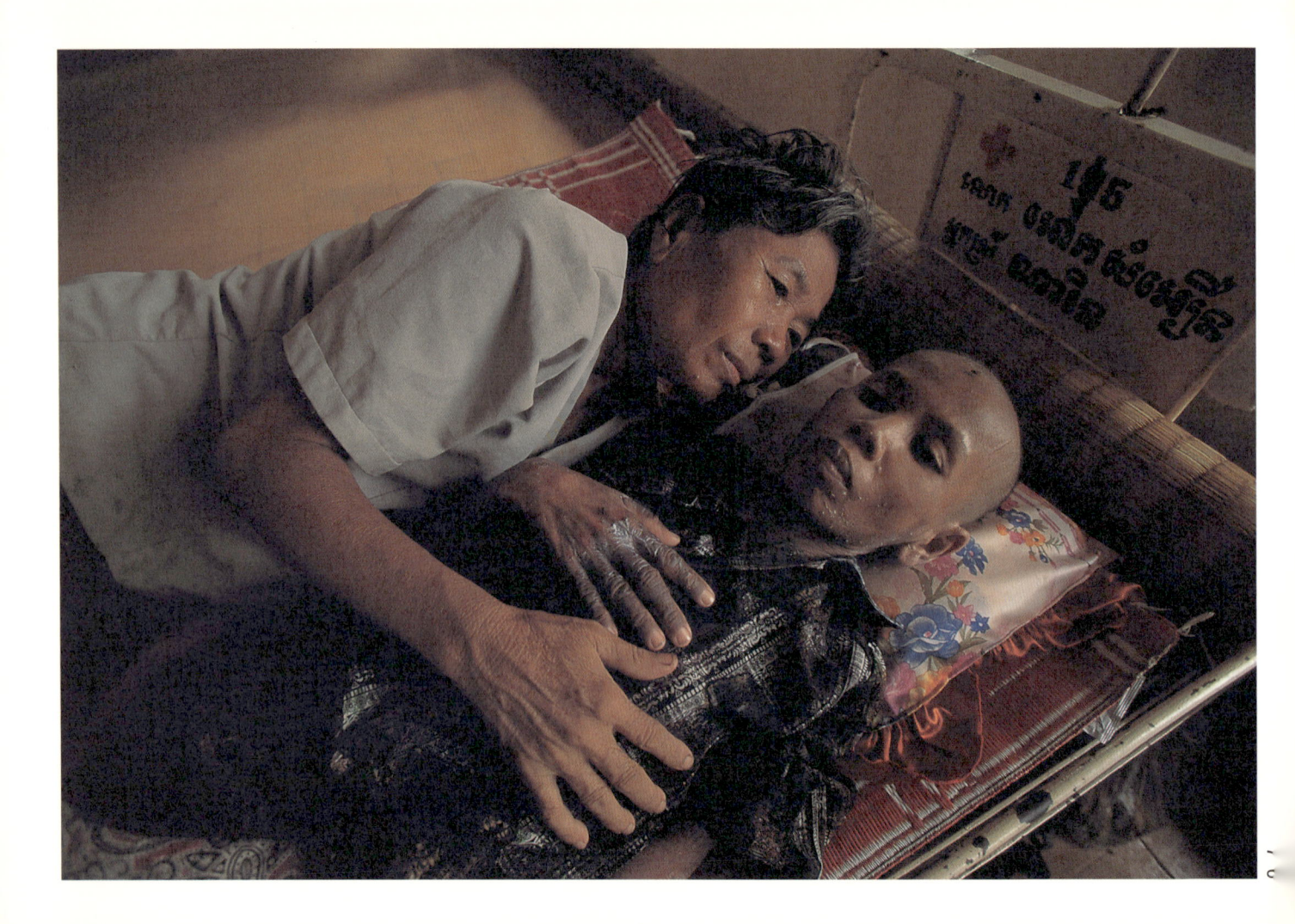

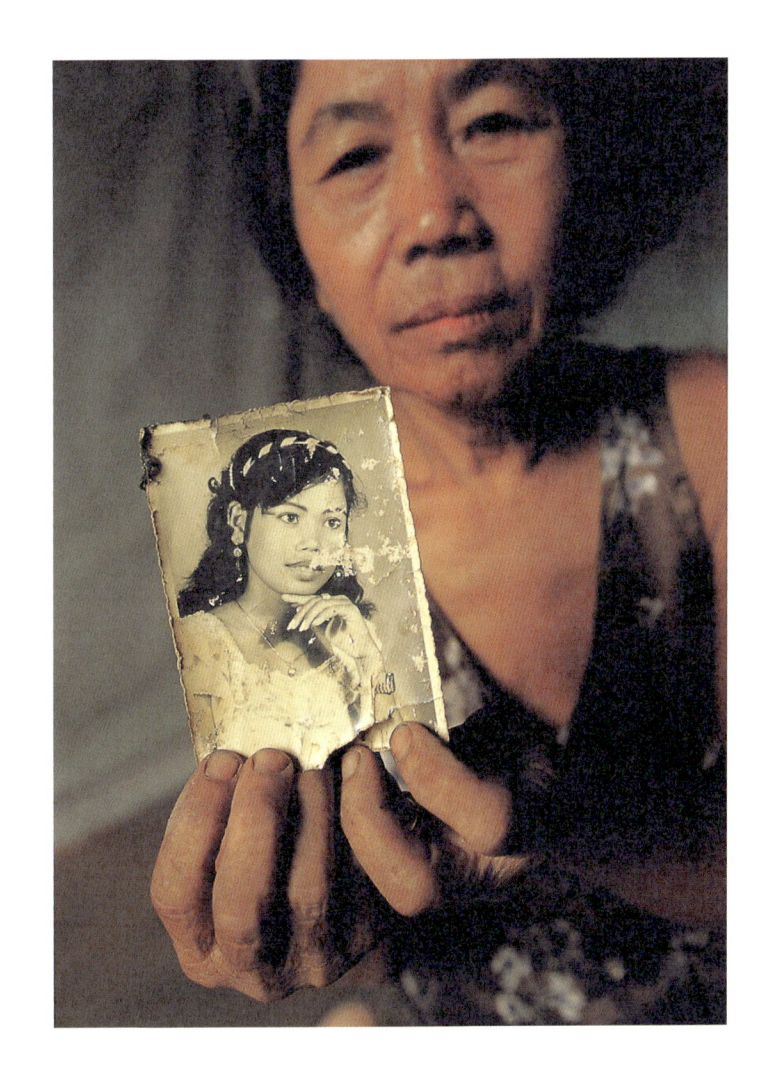

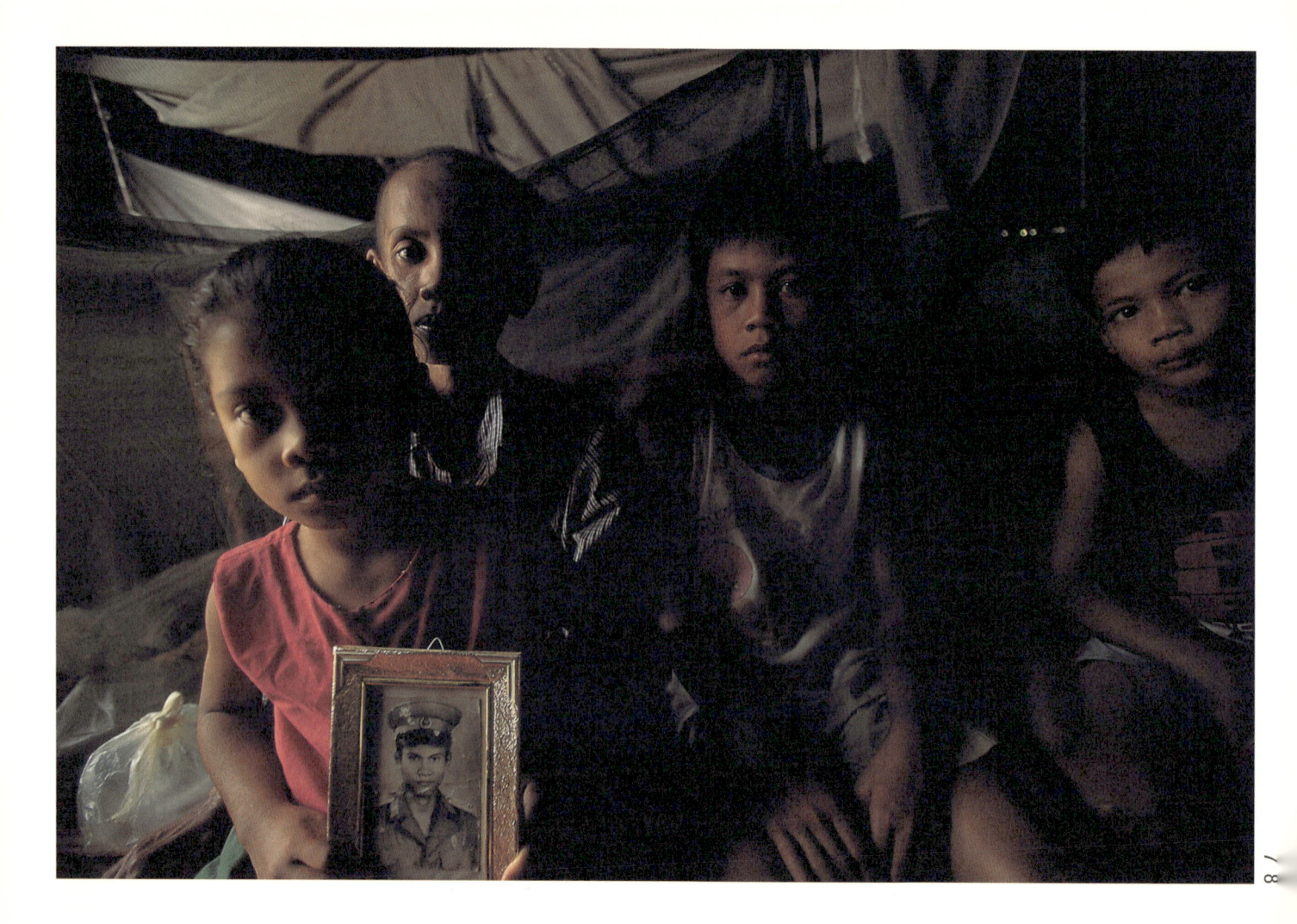

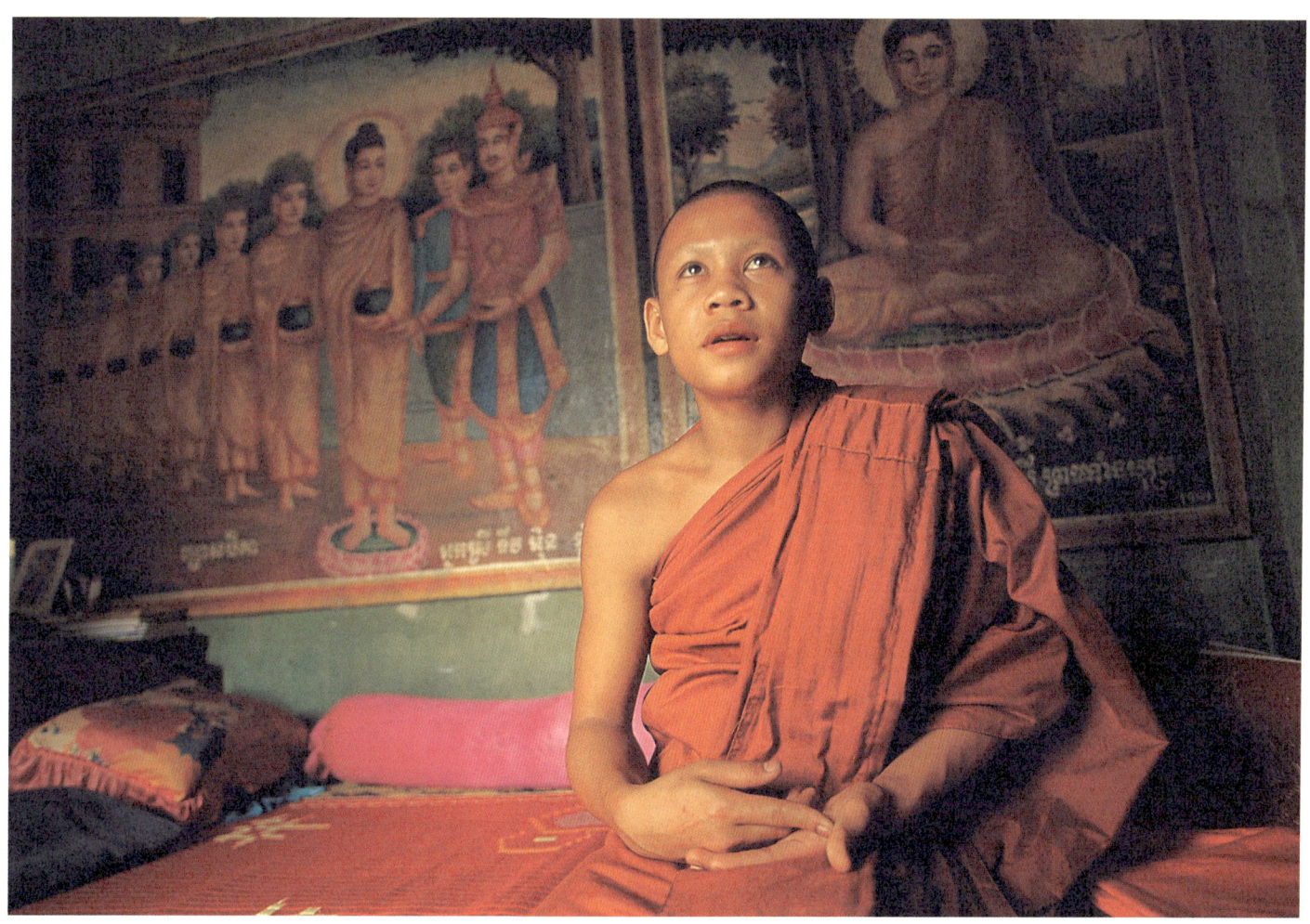

18 ホーン

　国立エイズ局によると、現在カンボジア国内のHIV感染者は16万人と言われ、そのうちエイズを発症している2万2000人が延命薬を必要としている。だが、保健省には約2700人分の薬しかなく、現在外国の援助団体の支援によって、首都プノンペンとシエムリアップ州にある3ヵ所の病院で約1000人分の延命薬が無料配給されている。といっても、くじ引きである。患者たちは数万人の登録者の中からくじ引きで薬をもらうのである。

　2004年5月。プノンペンで暮らす27歳のホーンと出会った。夫婦でエイズと判明したのは1998年だった。藁をもつかむ思いで地元の団体に相談すると、「一緒に働かないか」と誘われた。担当はエイズ教育で、彼女は自らの経験を話し、人々にエイズ予防を呼びかけた。そして翌年には運よく延命薬をもらう権利を得た。

　今、ホーンは夫と共にエイズの発症を抑える延命薬を飲んでいる。彼女は言う。

　「貧しくても、このままずっと家族と一緒に暮らしたい。そして、エイズ患者たちみなが、早く薬をもらえることを祈っています」

18 Horn

According to the National Aids Authority, there are 160,000 HIV patients in Cambodia, and among those patients, 22,000 need life-sustaining drugs. The Ministry of Health has these drugs, but only for 2,700 people. Now, a life-sustaining drug for about 1,000 people is distributed free through three hospitals in Phnom Penh and Siem Reap provinces, by a foreign aid group. But patients must be lucky to get the drugs, as they are distributed by lottery from perhaps one hundred thousand registrants.

In March 2004, I met Horn, 27, who lives in Phnom Penh. She and her husband found out in 1998 that they were HIV positive. When she visited a local organization to talk about her problem, they invited her to become an educator for them. She took charge of AIDS education for the group, and she talked about her personal experiences and appealed for AIDS prevention. The next year she had more good luck: she hit the lottery for life-sustaining drugs.

Now she and her husband are taking drugs to suppress HIV. "Even if we are poor, I want to live with my family all the time. And, I am praying that all AIDS patients will get medicine as soon as possible," she says.

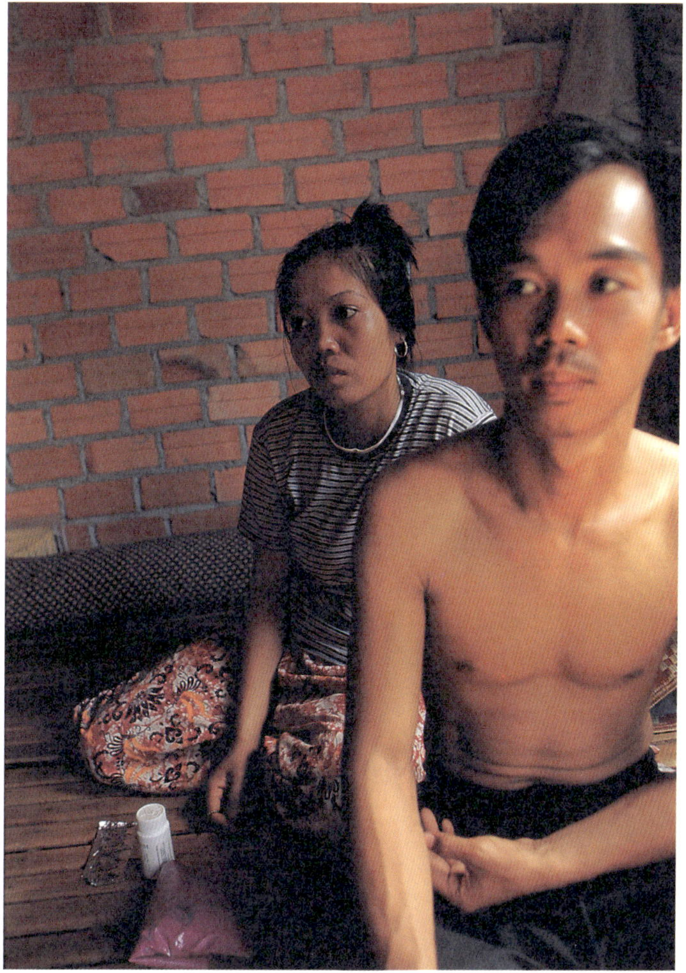

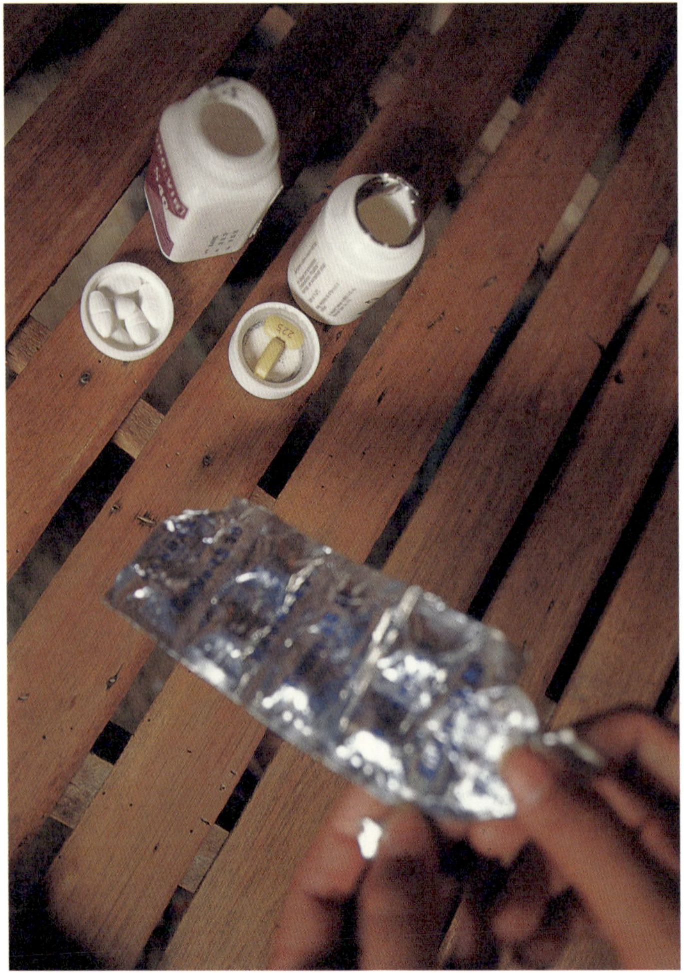

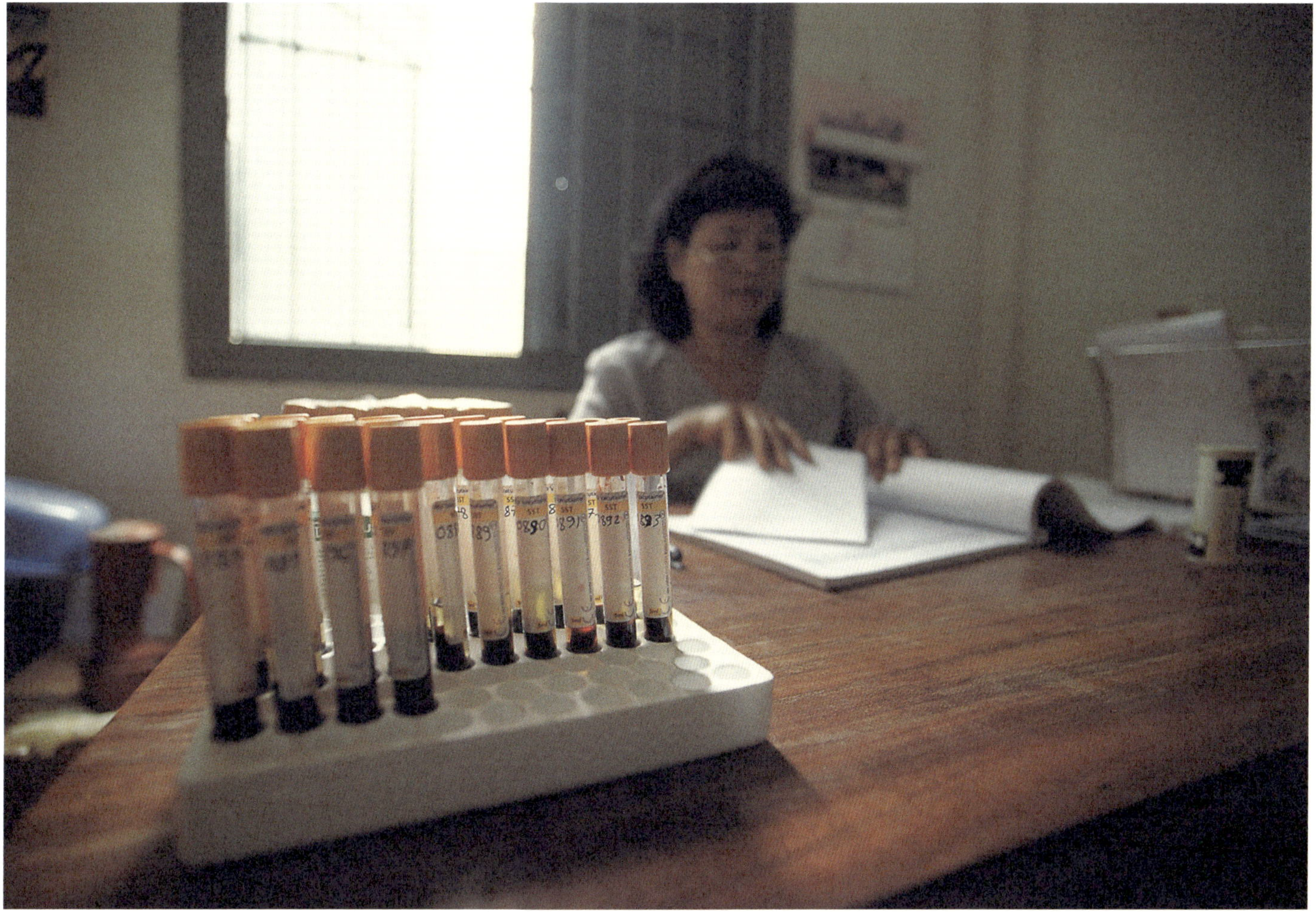

19 キーロック

　2004年5月。バッタンバン州のボウバル地区にあるクロス寺院には、エイズ患者の為のメディテイション・センターがある。施設は藁葺きや竹などで建てられたシンプルなものだ。ここで暮らす患者たちは、仏教の教えを学びながら、カンボジアの伝統生薬を飲んで養生している。クルー・クマエという生薬を作る専門の人がいて（クルーは先生、クマエはカンボジアの意味）、毎朝木々を細かく砕き、それを乾燥させて生薬を作っている。

　エイズ患者たちの中には、絶望して自ら命を絶つ者もいる。施設では夕方、僧侶が患者たちに仏教の教えを説く。

　「死を恐れてはいけません。死ぬことは自然なのです。すべてを受け入れなさい」

　ここではみな、助け合いながら生きている。運営しているティーン・トー・アソシエイション（TTA）代表のキーロックが言う。

　「もちろん、エイズのための高価な薬も必要です。しかし、他人を思いやること。その気持ちが何よりも大切なのです」

19　Ky Lok

　In May 2004, there is a meditation center for AIDS patients in the Kross temple of Bowbal district in Battambang province. The facilities are simple, built with straw and bamboo. The patients who live here are learning Buddhist instruction and they take a Cambodian traditional herb medicine for treatment. A special person, called Kru Khmer (Kru means teacher, Khmer means Cambodian), makes the herbal medicine. He cuts and grinds different types of wood every morning and makes the medicine by drying them.

　Among the AIDS patients there are some who killed themselves from despair. In the meditation center, a monk explains the tenets of Buddhism to the patients every evening.

　"You must not be afraid of death. Dying is natural. You must accept all."

　In the meditation center, all patients live by helping each other. Mr. Ky Lok is a representative of the Tean Thor Association (TTA) which manages the meditation center. He says, "Of course expensive medicine is necessary for AIDS patients, too. But, be considerate of other people. That feeling is the most important."

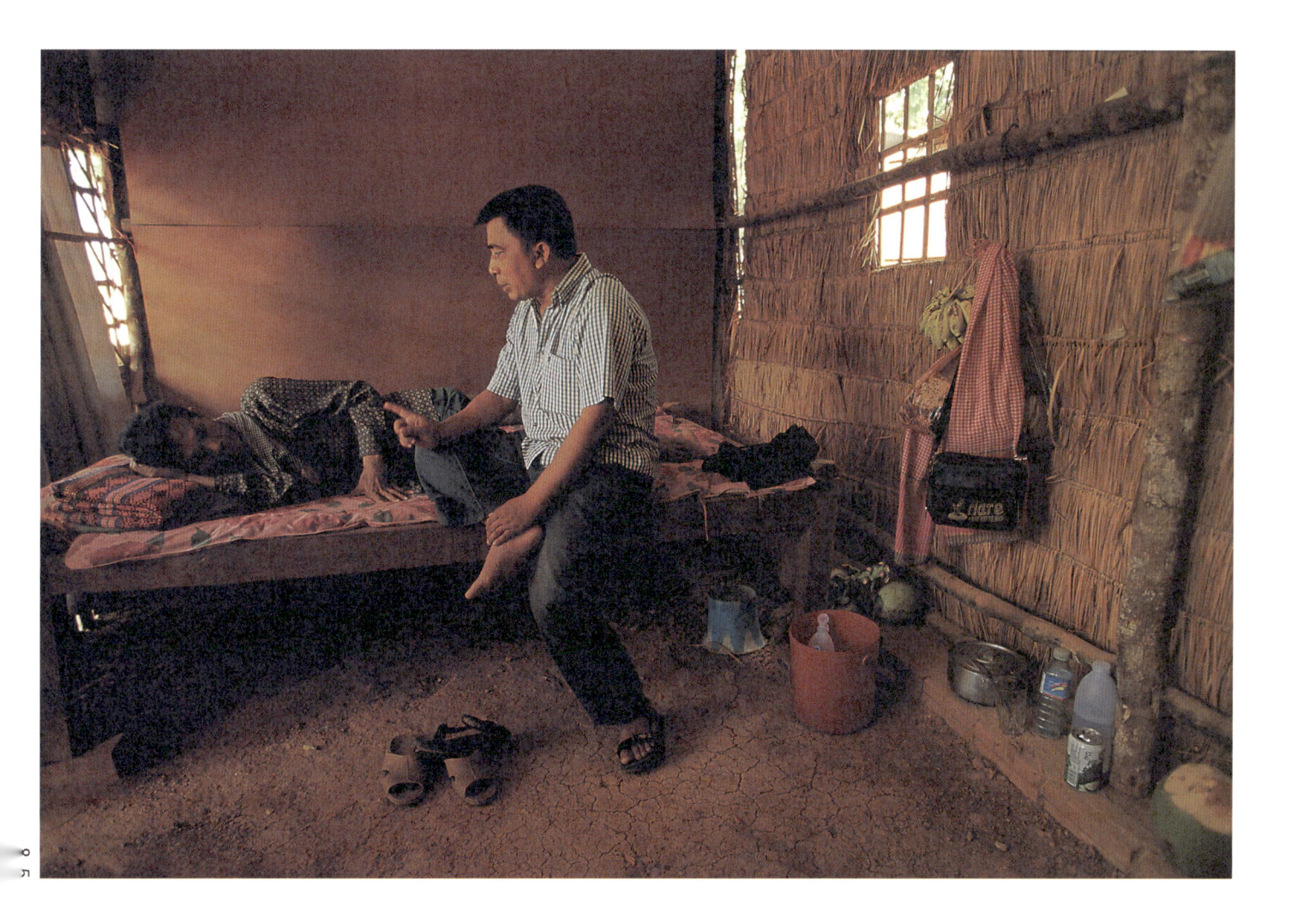

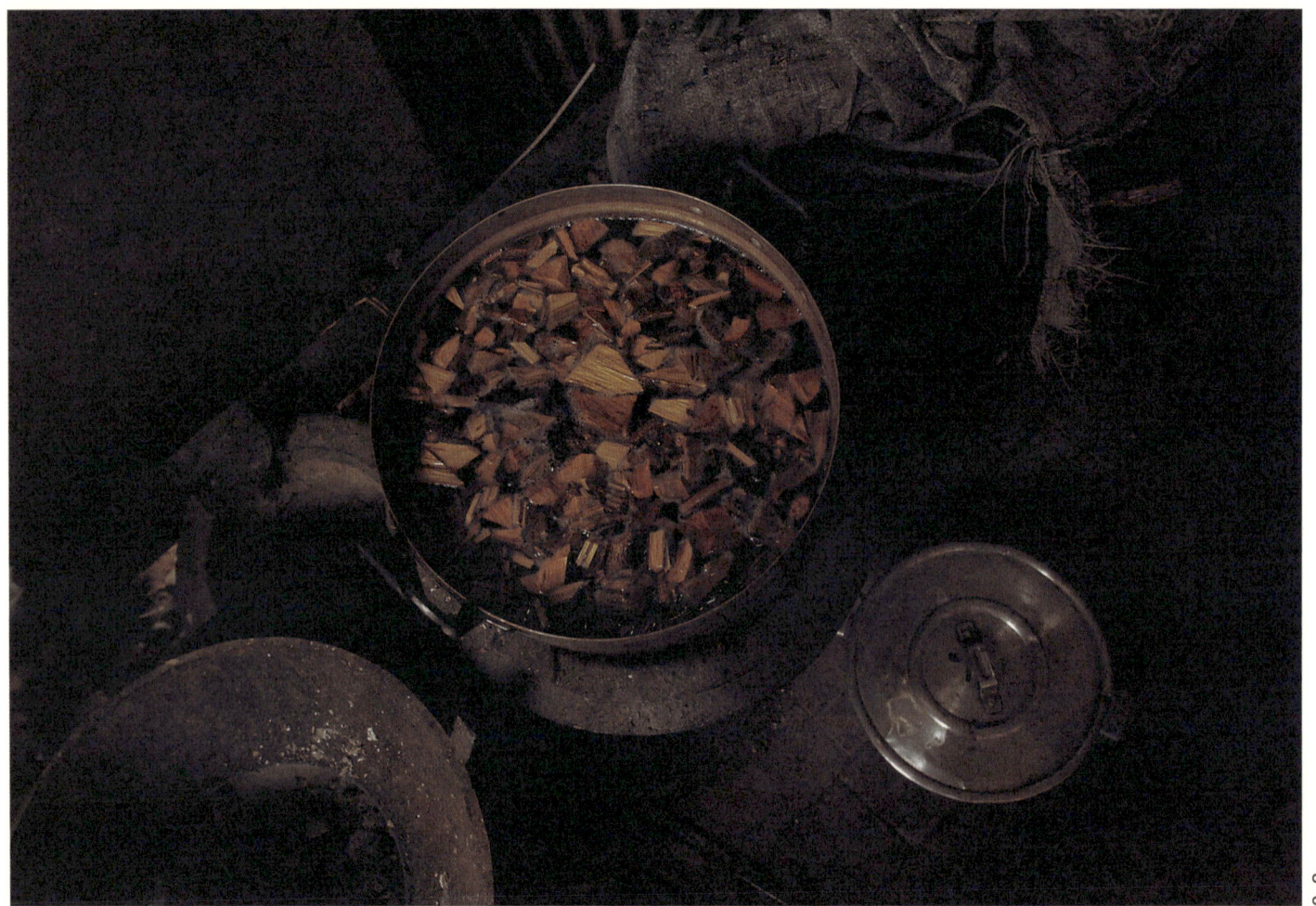

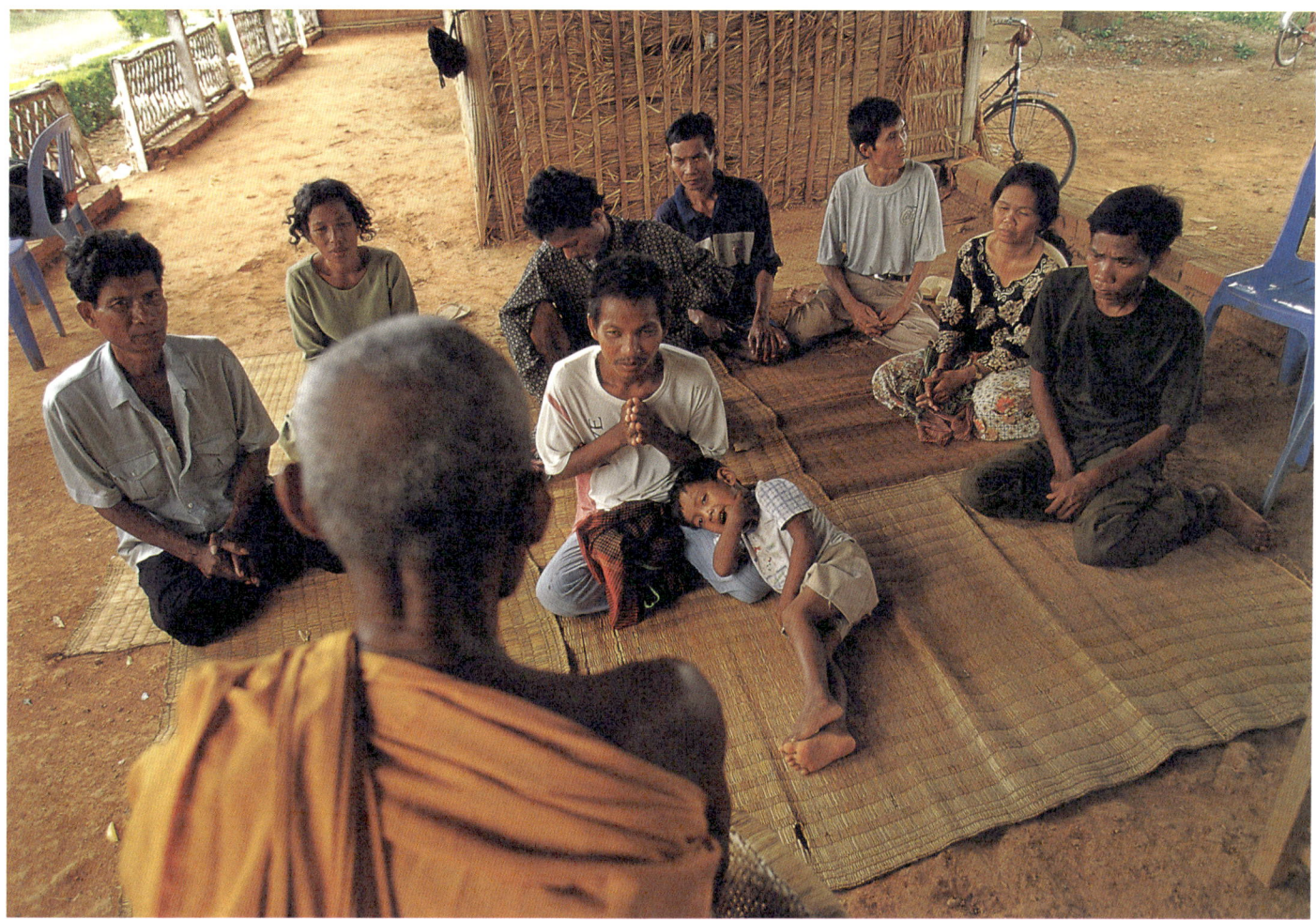

20　ティー

　2001年3月。小柄な女性がベッドに腰掛けていた。目が合うとニコッと笑い、彼女は言った。
　「私はティーよ。退屈だわ。ここに座ってお茶でも飲みませんか」
　壊れかけたベッドの隅に座ると、彼女は使い古されたアルミ製のヤカンから、朝淹れたというお茶をコップに注いでくれた。
　ひとり娘は祖父に預けてあるという。夫は1年ほど前、エイズで死んだ。
　「生きていてほしかった。でも夫が死んだ時、少し気持ちが楽になりました。闘病中、早く死にたい、殺してくれと、私に何度も言っていたから」
　以来ティーと会うたびに、色々な話をした。
　2002年5月、「記念撮影をして」と頼まれた。彼女はきれいにお化粧をして、一番大切な服を着ていた。彼女はいつもの笑顔で言った。
　「エイズをうつした夫を、私は恨んでいないわ。今私にできることは、毎日一生懸命生きることだけ」
　そして2ヵ月後、ティーはこの世を去った。

20　Tee

In March 2001, there is a small woman sitting on a bed in the epidemic ward. When I meet her gaze, she laughs with a charming smile, and she says, "I am Tee. I am bored. Would you like to sit here and drink some tea?"

When I sat on the corner of her bed, it began to break. Even so, she picked up a worn aluminum kettle and she poured her morning tea into a glass for me. She had sent her only daughter to her grandfather to take care of him. Her husband died from AIDS about a year before.

"I wanted him to live. But when my husband died, I felt some release. During his fight with AIDS, he said to me many times, 'I want to die, kill me now.'"

Since then, whenever I met Tee, we talked together about various things. One day she asked to me to "take my picture for memory." So she made herself up beautifully and wore her favorite clothes. She said with the usual smile, "I don't have any grudge against my husband who infected me with AIDS. Now all I can do is live very hard each day."

Then, two months later, Tee passed from this world.

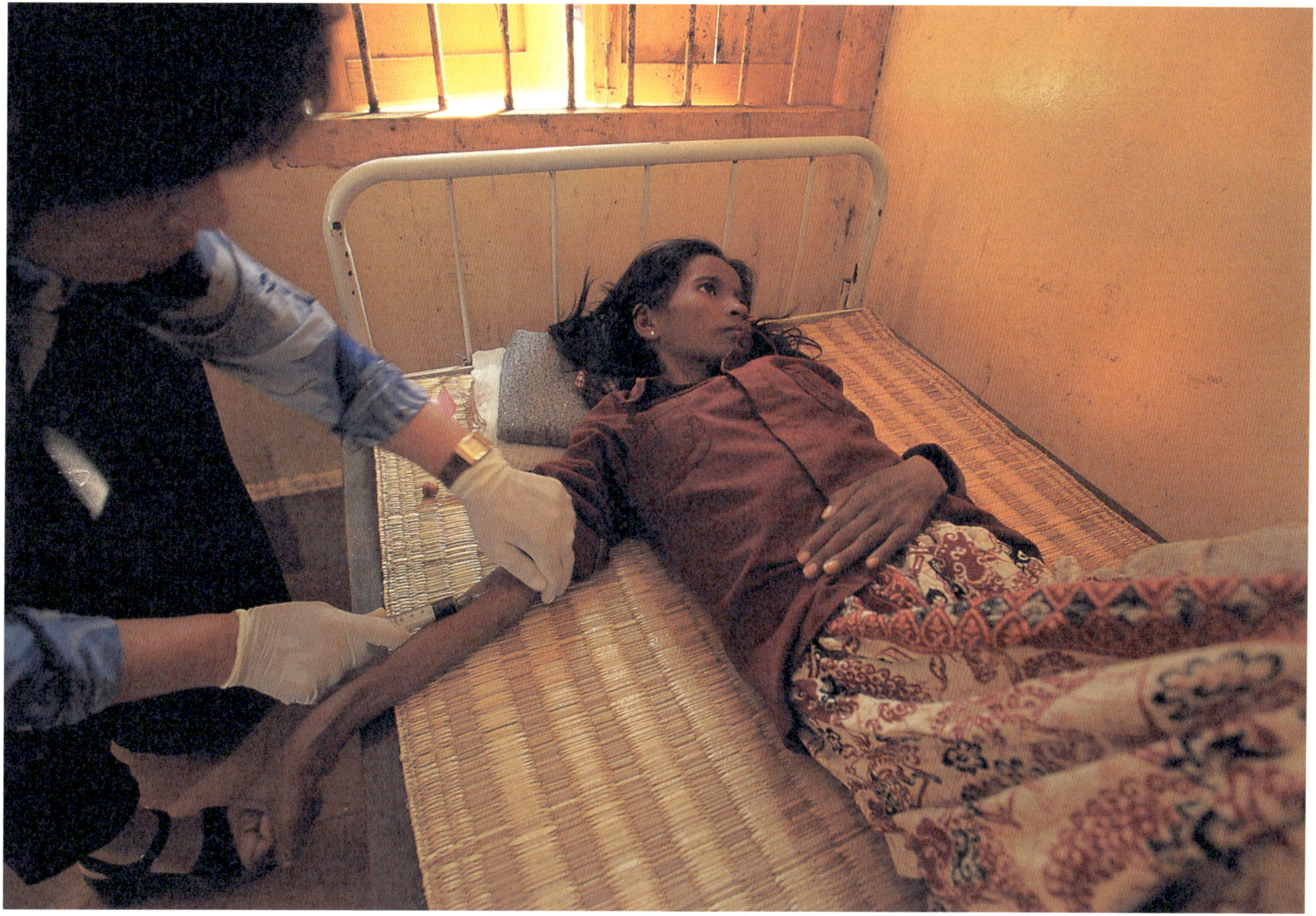

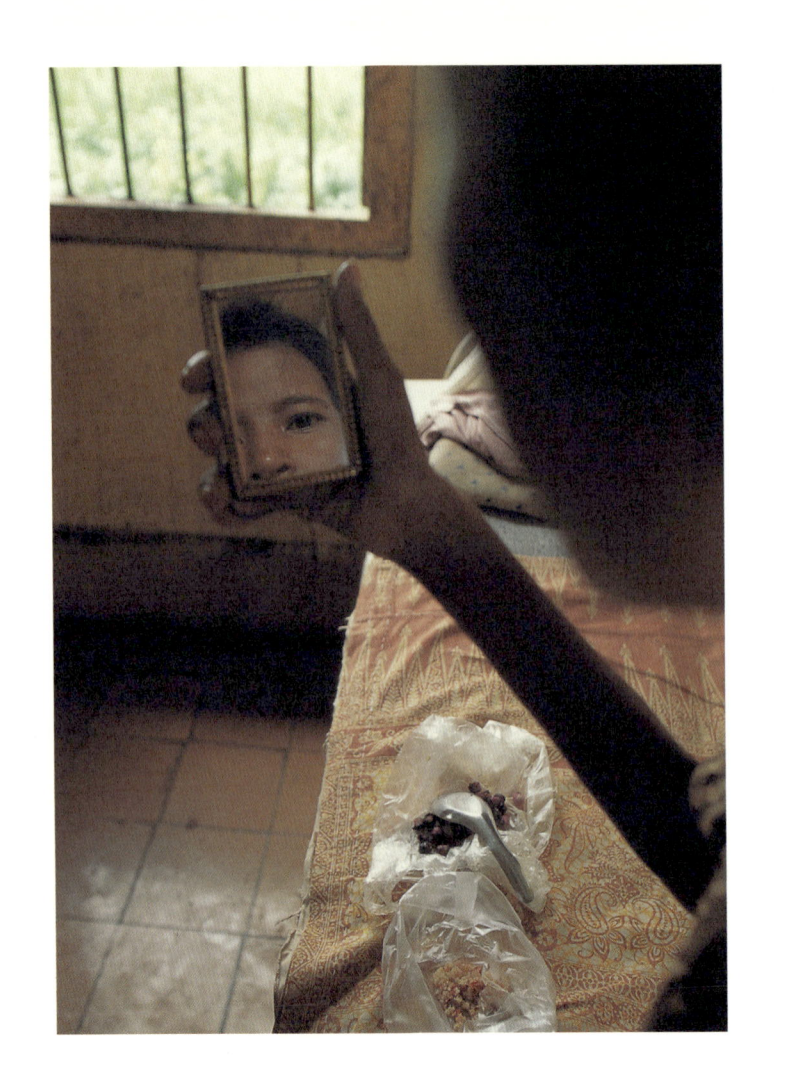

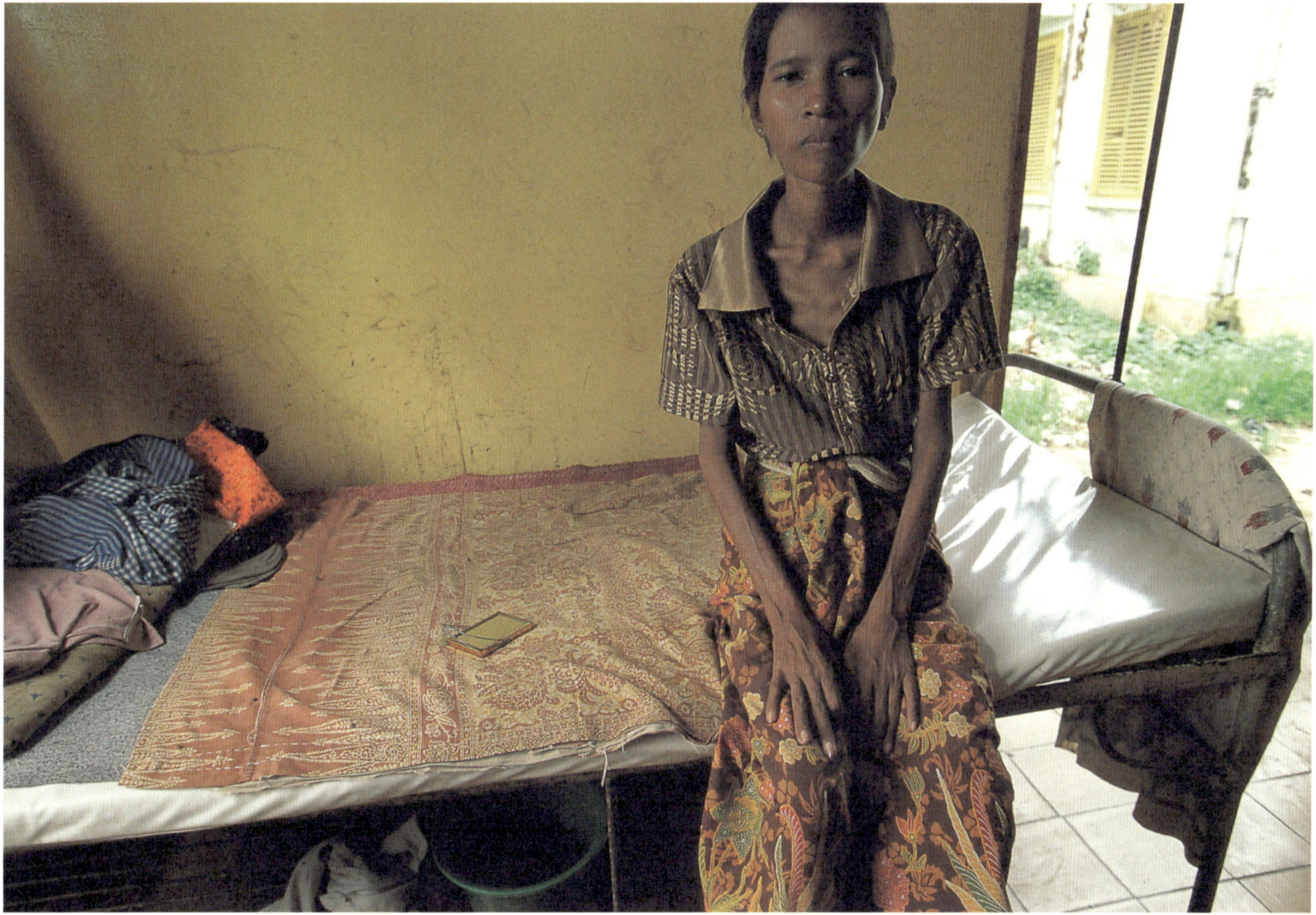

01

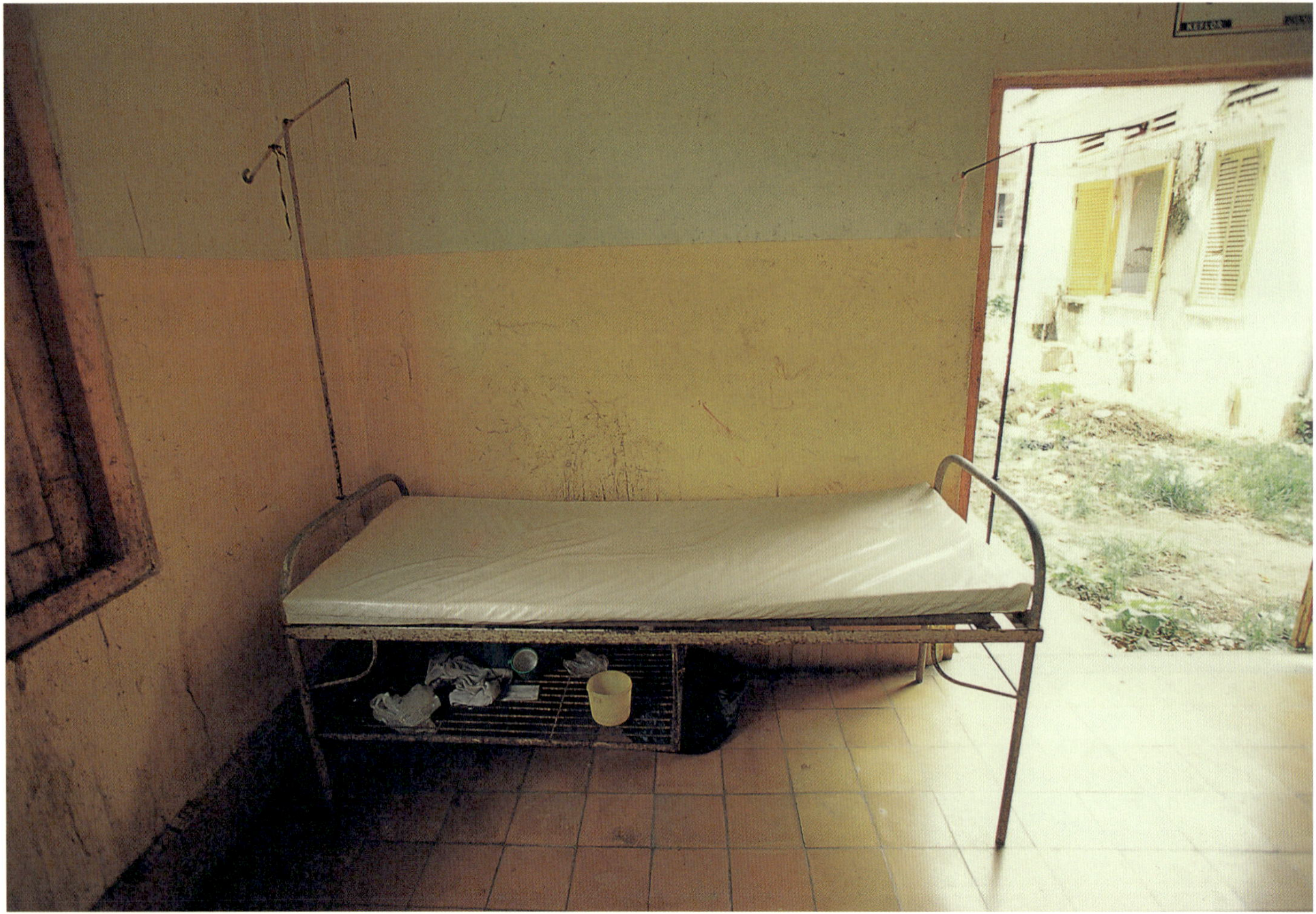

あとがき

　カンボジアのバッタンバン州はタイ国境に面している。人口およそ40万人。国内でも有数の米の産地で、郊外に一歩出ると、なだらかな平地がどこまでも続いている。
　1994年に初めてバッタンバンを訪れた僕は、前線で戦う少年兵や家を追われた難民たちの姿をカメラで追った。当時、カンボジアは内戦で国中がめちゃめちゃになっていた。バッタンバンは特に戦闘が激しく、毎年乾季になると大攻勢が始まり、病院は地雷や戦闘で傷ついた人々でいっぱいになった。病棟では、低いうめき声と悲痛な泣き声が絶えず響いていた。
　2001年、内戦が終わり、カンボジアにも平和が訪れたように見えた。しかし久しぶりにバッタンバンの病院を訪れた僕は啞然とした。やせ細って、枯れ木のようになった人々が病室に溢れている。ベッドが足りないらしく、床に寝ている者も多かった。患者たちは貧しく、持ち物はゴザと着替えぐらいで、みな食べる物さえ困っていた。
　「見てください。エイズという第2の内戦が、カンボジアを襲っているのです」
　感染病棟所長のスセップ医師が言った。骨と皮だけになった1人の女性患者の診察を終えた彼は、ポケットから少々のお金を出し、彼女にそっと渡した。
　「彼女は一銭も持っていない。患者たちはみな、苦しんでいる。このままでは、ここにいる全員が死んでしまいます」
　医師も看護師もみな、患者を助けたいという強い思いを抱いていた。しかし医療器具は古く、病院の設備も乏しかった。内戦中バッタンバンは情勢が不安定で、そのため第2の都市にもかかわらず、復興が随分と遅れていた。スセップ医師が寂しそうに言う。
　「2ヵ月間入院して、それでも症状が良くならなかったら、家に帰りなさいと患者たちに告げています。1人で死を迎えるより、家に帰り愛する家族にみとられながら死を迎えることを勧めているのです」
　カンボジアでは、エイズで苦しんでいる人々の多くが貧困層である。その後、僕は、売られたあとエイズを発症して死を迎える女性たちに数え切れないほど出会うことになった。カンボジアは確かに平和になった。しかし、国境にはカジノが建設され、売春街が巨大化し、ドラッグや児童売買などが公然と行なわれている。教育が行き届いていない農村地帯では、たやすく人身売買組織に騙されてしまう例が後を絶たない。今でも1ヵ月に400人から800人の子供たちが国外へ売られている。また、先進国では普通に買えるエイズ発症を抑える薬も、カンボジアの多くの人々には高価で手が届かない。広がる貧富の差と無秩序に発展した性産業。それがカンボジアにエイズを爆発的に蔓延させた最大の原因である。
　エイズで力尽きて死んでいく人々を目の当たりにすると、彼らの姿を記録しても無駄かもしれないと感じる時がある。でも僕にできることは、言葉にすることのできない人々の姿を記録し続けることしかない。彼らの姿を1人でも多くの人に見てもらい、そしてこの問題を一緒になって考えてもらうことが、患者たちの過酷な現状を変える第1歩になると思っている。
　写真は時に、非常に繊細な部分まで写しこむ。エイズ患者の悲惨な場面ばかり写しているという批判もあった。しかし、患者たちはみな、誰にも知られずに死んでゆくよりも、「私たちの存在」を人々に知らせたいと本気で願っていたことを書き留めておきたい。
　厳しい状況の中で僕を受け入れてくれたエイズと闘っている人たちに、心から敬意を示したい。

　このプロジェクトは人々の協力なしでは続けられなかった。マック・スセップ医師、ジニー・ハラシー（タイ外国人記者クラブ）、チャー・ピセ、ピーター・チャールスワースとイバン・コーヘン（オンアジア・イメージス）、高野佳雄さんと森山園生さん（元国際交流基金バンコック）、八鍬俊幸社長とスタッフの方々（エプソン・タイランド）、大江浩さんとスタッフの方々（横浜YMCA）、奥平亨さんと中村紀子さん（紀伊國屋書店）。英訳のコレクションを引き受けてくれたジェリー・レッドフェンとカレン・コート。リマインダーズ・プロジェクトの友人たち。良き理解者である朝日新聞社の朝日教之さん。いつも励ましてくれた母と兄。僕を支え続けてくれている妻の由美。そして最後に、この本の出版の機会を与えてくれためこんの桑原晨社長。1人1人に、本当に感謝します。ありがとう。

　この本は、フォトジャーナリストが現場の状況を伝えるために、そこに暮らす人々をテーマにしたものであり、被写体の人々の理解があった上で写真を掲載したことを記しておきたい

2005年3月、バンコックにて　　　後藤　勝

Epilogue

Cambodia's Battambang province faces the Thai border.

About 400,000 people live there. The province produces some of the country's best rice, and the grand, green scene spreads out on level ground in every direction outside Battambang town.

I first visited Battambang in 1994, and I turned my camera to the refugees who had left their villages, and to the child soldiers who fought on the front lines in the civil war.

At that time, Cambodia was ravaged by fighting. This was especially so in Battambang province, where people often found the front lines and heavy fighting just outside their front doors. Every year in the dry season, a big military offensive would begin, and Battambang hospital would fill with the people who were injured by land mines or crossfire. In the hospital wards, I always heard people crying and groaning.

In 2001, after the civil war ended, Cambodia seemed to be a peaceful country. But when I visited the Battambang hospital again, I was so surprised. The ward was full of patients who had become very thin, just like dead trees. The hospital seemed to be short of beds, and there were many patients sleeping on the floor.

All the patients were poor, and their belongings were only traditional thin mats and a few clothes. Food was a problem for many patients because few of them had any money.

"Please look at this," said Dr. Sutthep, the chief of the epidemic ward at the hospital. "AIDS, Cambodia's second civil war, is attacking now."

When he finished the medical examination of one woman who was only bone and skin, he took a little money from his pocket and gave it to her gently. "She doesn't have any money. All the patients are suffering. Without any treatment, all of them will die soon."

The thought to help the patients was common to the doctor and his nurses. But the hospital's medical equipment was old and in poor condition. The situation was unstable in Battambang during the civil war. Even though this is Cambodia's second-largest city, reconstruction has been very slow. And there is very little to help the patients in the epidemic ward.

"If a symptom doesn't improve within two months, I tell the patient to go back to their home," Dr. Sutthep said sorrowfully. "Because rather than die alone, a family who loves them can nurse them until they pass away. That's what I advise them."

Most of the people suffering from AIDS in Cambodia are poor. I have seen innumerable women who were sold to human traffickers because of poverty, and then they died of AIDS.

Cambodia became peaceful after its civil war ended. But in the border area between Cambodia and Thailand, many casinos have been built, and a prostitution town has grown. The drug trade and child trafficking are done openly, if not exactly legally. The education system does not reach the rural areas, so people there are often easily deceived by human traffickers. Even now, in one month, between 400 and 800 Cambodian children are sold to foreign countries through human traffickers.

People can get anti-retroviral medicines to fight AIDS in advanced countries. But most Cambodians are not able to buy these medicines because they are too expensive. The sex industry developed explosively as the gap between rich and poor widened, and this further spread AIDS in Cambodia.

When I see patients dying with AIDS, I sometimes feel that taking their picture is not very helpful.

But all I can do is take pictures of the patients and their families. They are voiceless, and I hope that many people will see their photos and hear their stories. I want people to think about this problem together. I believe that it will be one step on the road to changing the severe present condition of AIDS patients in Cambodia.

These pictures sometimes show very delicate moments. Some people have criticized these images because they felt despair. They said that these images are only tragic scenes of AIDS patients.

But I want to write down that all of the patients sincerely wanted to tell the world about their lives, rather than dying in silence. I want show my huge respect for the people who fight AIDS and welcomed me into their lives, even in their most severe moments.

I could not continue this project without the continued cooperation and help from these people: Doctor Sutthep, Jeanne Hallacy of The Foreign Correspondents Club of Thailand, Chath Piseth, Peter Charlesworth and Yvan Cohen of OnAsia Images, Mr. Takano, Ms. Moriyama of The Japan Foundation Bangkok, Mr. Yakuwa, President of Epson Thailand, and his staff, Mr. Ohe and staff of the Yokohama YMCA, Mr. Okudaira and Mrs. Nakamura of the KINOKUNIYA BOOK STORE. Jerry Redfern and Karen Coates helped with the English translations in this book. Friends of Reminder's Project. I thank Mr. Noriyuki Asahi at Asahi News Paper for his understanding in this project. My mother and brother always encouraged me. And my wife Yumi has always supported me. And last but not least, president of Mekong Publishing, Mr. Kuwahara, gave me a chance to publish this book.

I really appreciate each person. Thank you.

Masaru Goto, Maroh 2005

"This book is to introduce the world to the situation of HIV/AIDS in Cambodia. The theme is the people who live there, and each photo was made with the understanding and cooperation of the people shown."

Special thanks to
Battambang province
Battambang Referral Hospital
Battambang Military Hospital
Bawbal district Hospital
Sudau district clinic
Pailin Hospital
Chivith Mey (New Life)
Cambodian Women for Peace and Development (CWPD)
Reproductive Health Association of Cambodia (RTTA)
Cambodian Health Education Development (CHED)
Komar Rik Reay Association Center
Vocational Training Center Battambang
Emergency (Surgical Center for War Victims)
World Vision Cambodia
League of Cambodian Journalists (LCJ)
Operations Enfants de Battambang (O.E.B)
Trauma Care Foundation
Battambang Women's Aids Project (BWAP)
Cambodian Women for Peace and Development (CWPD)

Siem Reap province
Siem Reap Province Hospital
Siem Reap Military Hospital
Leucaena Communication Japonesia

Banteay Meanchey province
Enfants du Mekong
Krousar Thmey
Associations pour la Development Technique de la Jeunesse Khmer

Phnom Penh
Sihanouk Hospital
Calmette Hospital
Family Health International (FHI)
Pact Cambodia
Oxfam
Mith Samlanh (Friends)

Cambodian Women's Crisis Center
Sacrifice Family and Orphans Development Association (SFODA)
Cambodian League for the Promotion and Defense of Human Rights (LICADHO)
Urban Sector Group (USG)
Cambodian Light Children and Orphan Training Center (C.L.C.A)
Vulnerable Children Assistance Organization (VCAO)
Cambodian Disabled Independent Living Organization (CDILO)
Transcultural Psychosocial Organization (TPO)
Cambodian People Living With HIV/AIDS Network (CPN)
Reproductive and Child Health Alliance (RACHA)
National Aids Authority
UN Volunteers
Hope world wide
Khemara
The World Bank
Reuters Phnom Penh
Associated Press Phnom Penh
Deutsche Presse Agentur GmbH (DPA)
Phnom Penh Post
The Cambodia Daily

Bangkok
OnAsia Images
Action Aid Thailand
Joint United Nations Programme on HIV/AIDS (UNAIDS)
United Nations Children's Found (UNICEF THAILAND)
Economic and Social Commission for Asia and the Pacific (UNESCAP)
Asian Forum for Human Rights and Development (FORUM ASIA)
Empower Foundation
Life Home Project
Epson Thailand
The Japan Foundation Bangkok
The Foreign Correspondents Club of Thailand (FCCT)

後藤勝（ごとう　まさる）　1966年生まれ。名古屋市出身。高校中退後アメリカに渡る。中南米を放浪後、1992年から南米コロンビアの人権擁護団体と活動する。現在はバンコクを拠点にし、フォトジャーナリストとしてアジアの人権問題を追う。オンアジア・イメージス所属。
E-mail　masarugoto1@mail.goo.ne.jp

受賞歴
2004年　第5回上野彦馬賞（九州産業大学、毎日新聞社）
2004年　"The River of Life" 国際写真コンペティション（世界保健機関）
2002年　"The Photo Fund 2002" International Fund for Documentary Photography Fifty Crows Foundation

著書　『カンボジア・僕の戦場日記』（めこん、1999年）
共著　『ジャーナリズムの条件1』『職業としてのジャーナリスト』（筑紫哲也編、岩波書店、2005年）

Profile
Masaru Goto was born in Nagoya City, Japan, in 1966. After dropping out of high school, he moved to the United States. In 1992, he started work as a photojournalist in South America, with a human rights group in Colombia. He currently focuses on human rights issues in Asia. He is a member of On Asia Images in Bangkok.
E-mail　masarugoto1@mail.goo.ne.jp

Awards
2004
"Ueno Hikoma Award"
Kyushu Sangyo University, Mainichi Newspaper
2004
"The River of Life" International Photo Competition
Won two categories, "LOVE" and "ILLNESS"
World Health Organization (WHO)
2002
"The Photo Fund 2002"
International Fund for Documentary Photography
Fifty Crows Foundation

Publications
"My Journal in Cambodia."
Mekong publishing,Tokyo,1999

絶望のなかのほほえみ——カンボジアのエイズ病棟から

初版第1刷　2005年4月30日

定価　2000円＋税

著者　後藤勝
装丁　菊地信義
発行者　桑原晨
発行　株式会社めこん
〒113-0033　東京都文京区本郷3-7-1
電話03-3815-1688　FAX03-3815-1810
URL http://www.mekong-publishing.com

印刷・製本　ローヤル企画
0030-0503182-8347

ISBN4-8396-0182-8 C0030 ¥2000E

©2005, Goto　Masaru, Printed in Japan